FINDING TRUTH
IN
TRANSPARENCY

About the Author

Dr. Paul David Rocky Bilhartz is a graduate of Rice University. He received a joint Medical Doctor (M.D.) and Master of Business Administration (M.B.A.) degree with specialization in Health Organizational Management from Texas Tech University Health Science Center in Lubbock, Texas. He completed his residency in Internal Medicine, fellowship in Cardiovascular Disease, and subspecialty fellowship in Interventional Cardiology at Texas A&M University Health Science Center, Scott & White Memorial Hospital, in Temple, Texas. During this time, he was chosen as Intern of the Year, elected to Alpha Omega Alpha Honor Medical Society, and received the C. Charles Welch Scott & White Hospital Outstanding Resident Award.

Dr. Bilhartz currently operates his own private practice in Interventional Cardiology & Cardiovascular Disease and serves as a Clinical Assistant Professor at Texas A&M Health Science Center School of Medicine. He is the developer of ECGsource.com, an online cardiovascular medical education resource, and he is the creator of three mobile medical education applications (ECGsource, CathSource, and EchoSource), which are available for both the iPhone and Android Operating Systems. He has been named to the Texas Super Doctors 2014 Rising Stars List in Texas Monthly Magazine, and he is board certified in Interventional Cardiology, Cardiovascular Disease, Nuclear Cardiology, and Internal Medicine. Dr. Bilhartz is a Fellow in both the American College of Cardiology and the Society for Cardiovascular Angiography and Interventions. He resides in College Station, Texas, with his wife, Lindsey, and children, Preston and Peyton.

FINDING TRUTH IN TRANSPARENCY

Our Broken Healthcare System and How We Can Heal It

Rocky D. Bilhartz, MD, MBA

2014
GREEN PUBLISHING HOUSE, LLC
College Station, Texas

Dedication

To Lindsey Lee Barton Bilhartz, for loving you has always been as natural as breathing; and to our children, Preston Bradley and Peyton Ryan, whom I challenge to always "fill the unforgiving minute with sixty-seconds' worth of distant run[1]"

---

[1] This phrase is taken from arguably one of the most inspiration poems of all time, *If—*, written by British Nobel laureate Rudyard Kipling.

Table of Contents

Introduction

"THE PEOPLE WHO ARE CRAZY ENOUGH
TO THINK THEY CAN CHANGE THE
WORLD, ARE THE ONES WHO DO."[1]

Healthcare is as complex as ever, and in many ways, the system makes absolutely no sense anymore. Yet, if you are reading this in hopes that I have a perfect solution to its problems, you can put this book down. Return it and try to get your money back. If a solution were that easy, someone would have figured it out by now. The problems are hard ones to solve. Yes, I have some ideas that will leak out over the course of this book, but ultimately you are reading this book because, like me, you live for truth. You want to know what really happens in the back when you take your car to the dealership for repairs. You want to know why the guy fixing your septic system really needs all those parts. You want to know why you've heard that you should be skeptical of your doctor. You want to know what is really going on behind that seemingly closed door of healthcare. You wonder why your health insurance sucks, your bill is indecipherable, your appointment time is delayed, and your physician is frustrated with societal demands placed on him or her. You want answers, and trust me, if I knew anything about car dealerships or septic systems, I'd include that in this book too. But, I don't know about those things. What I do know, however, is lots about healthcare. In fact, that's why you opened this book, and if truth is what you seek, you will be extremely pleased that you did.

This book is far from one of complaints. I absolutely love my job, and I believe that I work in one of the most challenging and rewarding professions in the world. Notwithstanding, it's the only major profession that I've ever had, so I'm biased, but still honored and blessed to be a physician in the United States of America.

Your problem is that you believe healthcare is a right. Admit it. I know this for two reasons: (1) I see you, or someone like you, every day in my clinic whose actions toward my front desk staff are confirmatory, and (2) because I feel exactly the same way. In fact, healthcare should be added alongside our right to life, liberty, and the pursuit of happiness. We have a right to be healthy, and who can blame us. If we don't have our health, what do we really have? Illness. And, none of us want that.

Case in point. When was the last time you went to the home improvement store, filled your cart full of light bulbs, lumber, tools, paint, flowers, and a barbecue grill? Then, pushed the cart to the front, waved your hand at the cashier, and without paying a dime, loaded up your truck and drove off? Unless you are reading this in prison, I suspect that you haven't engaged in such a ritual. But, this is precisely how you really feel healthcare should be for you. How do I know this? Because we all feel that we are entitled to the best light bulbs, lumber, tools, paint, flowers, and grill that healthcare has to offer. $665 out-of-pocket weekly for some allergy shots? Are you kidding me? I deserve those things at cost, or better yet, free, at my scheduled appointment time, or any other time that I might want to swing by the clinic last minute when it's convenient for me.

This book is about transparency in healthcare, but why do we crave this transparency so much? That's easy. We have always sought transparency when (1) value is disputed, and (2) fraud is suspected. For example, we want our government to be transparent in times when we doubt its worth. We want our church to divulge its financial books when we fear internal embezzlement. And, if I can't see the value that you are providing, you must be cheating me, and I want to know how you are doing it. Truth is the only thing that sets us free.

Healthcare is no different. You dispute its value. And, why is that not surprising? Because, there can be no value in something that costs money when you think it should be free. You suspect fraud. Your bill is too high, your doctor is too rich, your insurance plan is too confusing, and your trust in the system is nowhere to be found. Contrast that to the amazing home improvement store around the corner from your neighborhood. This is your most valued weekend errand. You go pick out your garden plants and paint colors. The guy who co-founded the place is worth a mere $3.5 billion, which should entitle you to leave with the items in your cart for free, but you don't. In fact, you gladly pay for them. Not every time do you get the most expensive hammer, but you still leave happy with your purchase, because this man's store has value to you. You don't even think about that man, and his wealth, nor expect him to answer your call after hours when the store is closed. His own transparency never crosses your mind. It doesn't even seem applicable.

----

[1] This quote was first used in an Apple, Inc. television commercial narrated by Richard Dreyfuss. It was a part of the company's *Think Different* advertising campaign, which launched in 1997. The entire full version of the quote appears below and has often provided me inspiration: "Here's to the crazy ones. The misfits. The rebels. The troublemakers. The round pegs in the square holes. The ones who see things diffcrently. They're not fond of rules. And they have no respect for the status quo. You can quote them, disagree with them, glorify or vilify them. But the only thing you can't do is ignore them. Because they change things. They push the human race forward. And while some may see them as the crazy ones, we see genius. Because the people who are crazy enough to think they can change the world, are the ones who do."

CHAPTER 1:

Building Credibility

"HONESTY IS THE FIRST CHAPTER
IN THE BOOK OF WISDOM."
—THOMAS JEFFERSON

I am 37 years old. I am a private practice physician. This means that I'm not employed by a hospital or a healthcare institution. I work for myself. With the money that I collect, I pay myself, as well as three employees who work exclusively for me, with one of these employees dealing solely with the complexities of billing within our healthcare system. I also pay one-fourth of the salaries and benefits of 10 more people who collectively assist myself and the three other physicians with whom I share common office space. This group of shared full-time workers includes front desk staff, office managers, and trained technicians who perform our in-office testing.

My specialty is interventional cardiology and cardiovascular disease. This means that I'm a heart and blood vessel doctor trained not only to diagnose and medically treat illnesses, but also to perform certain invasive procedures when needed. You may have heard of heart stress tests, nuclear studies, and echocardiograms. You may have heard of ultrasound procedures of the neck or extremities for detecting blood flow abnormalities, or the aorta for detecting an aneurysm. You may yourself have even had a stent placed, which is best described as a small "pipe" that is used to open a blockage that exists in your heart, neck, or extremity. You may know a relative with a pacemaker. These are all some of the things that I do on a daily basis.

But, let's get back to talking about my private practice. I've been doing this now for just over 3 years. This was essentially my first "real" job. Much of the previous two decades in my life were spent training for this incredible opportunity. In fact, you'll get to learn more about my training in the pages to come, but let's focus on the financial aspects of my practice right now.

MY ANNUAL SALARY

At the time that I'm writing this, the median annual salary for an interventional cardiologist in the United States, according to Salary.com, is $380,000. This is a lot of money, and my own practice is somewhere within this ballpark figure. But, if that's all that I told you, this wouldn't even be close to a book about healthcare transparency. And, remember, it's only the truth that sets us free. Just as being in the ballpark won't cut it anymore, glazing the surface of a profession whose value is being challenged isn't going to shatter opinions. Digging deeper into the vault of healthcare is all but required.

I pay myself a salary of $300,000 per year. That's still a whole lot of money. To be honest, I'm not quite for sure why I'm below the median number in my specialty. Maybe, I can convince you that I'm just starting out in my profession, and that I'm still in the early years of building up my practice from scratch. Maybe, it's because it's much harder than it used to be to make a private practice work, supported by the recent trend for private practitioners to sell their practices in favor of an employed position with a large healthcare entity or hospital. Indeed, the major draw for a salaried position within a mega-institution is that you finally have a wall of protection between yourself and the so-called monsters who seem to constantly be changing the reimbursement rules to make it more difficult for you to survive on your own.

Honestly, I just hope that you won't view my comparative salary numbers as some indication that you get what you pay for and my quality is below the average. No, let's look at it for now as if I'm just providing you better overall *value*. Ultimately, I guess that you'd have to ask some of my patients to make sure.

Keep in mind, however, that my $300,000 annual salary is really a moving target that translates to an average monthly amount of $25,000. Some months have the potential to be better than average. Other months may be worse, especially if I take an entire week of vacation (although I haven't done that yet in my three years of practice), or there are less work days in a month such as February. As I write this, I'm completing my sixth month of the fiscal year. I was $7,000 behind for the first month and $6,000 under for the second. All that means is that I borrowed money from myself to pay myself. Collections picked up for whatever reason in months three through six, and I've finally made back all but $3,000 of the $13,000 that I borrowed over the first two months. If the next six months are a repeat of the previous, I'll end up being only $6,000 short of my anticipated $300,000 annual salary for this current year.

You should know that the majority of my salary is from revenue generated from patient care related issues. I do, however, earn other physician-related income that is included in (and not in addition to) my salary above. For example, last fiscal year, I was paid about $5,000 from the local medical school to participate in teaching some of its medical students. I also enjoy speaking, and I've accepted invitations to lecture as a consultant for several medical corporations (more explanation about this will come later). These additional hours of work, outside of my private practice clinical duties, have made up about 7% of my annual salary over the last two years.

PRIVATE PRACTICE OVERHEAD

When I established my private practice three years ago, the greatest learning experience that I initially encountered was gaining an understanding of my necessary overhead costs. In fact, my overhead costs are so unbelievably outrageous that you wouldn't believe them if I told you. But, if you've learned anything about me yet, you know that I'm about to share these figures with you anyway.

This past month I had my standard expenses. I paid my usual $6,000 for rent, $15,000 for employee salaries and benefits, $4,500 toward bank notes on various types of testing equipment that I use for patient care, $1,000 more for insurance and service contracts on this equipment, and then $10,000 on medical supplies needed for me to conduct my in-office testing. This latter number seems unbelievably high, but my medical supply list includes nuclear radioisotopes used for cardiac stress testing, and that isotope generator isn't available for purchase from just anyone. When you throw in my utilities, which include the necessary electricity required to run these ginormous in-office medical machines (side note: the local utility company brings my office large baskets of fruit for the holidays as a thank you for our business each year), the final monthly figure for baseline overhead costs, prior to paying myself a dollar, is about $50,000.

Usually, every month I will also have some once-yearly miscellaneous fees. Thankfully, for me, the one-time fees are usually spaced out throughout the year, so I don't have to pay them all in the same month. On average, there are about two miscellaneous fees that I will pay each month. For example, this past month, in addition to the $50,000 of standard expenses listed above, I paid another $11,000 toward my employees' retirement (401(k)) plans. Next month, my miscellaneous fees will include $5,000 for my medical malpractice insurance and $890 to renew my medical license. All told, in any given month, it is not uncommon for overhead to exceed $55,000. Anything that I collect beyond that begins to pay my own salary.

VACATION TIME

When you are in private practice, vacation time is always a conflicting endeavor. You obviously need time to break away temporarily from any profession in order to avoid burnout. However, your monthly bills (for example, employee salaries and benefits, rental space, equipment costs) are predominantly fixed costs. On vacation, you aren't generating any revenue for your practice, but your bills for that month are essentially the same. Practically speaking, one week of vacation every quarter (equivalent to four total vacation weeks per year), costs me an estimated $80,000 per year. Then, on top of that, you get to pay for the actual vacation, which ultimately results in you taking very few vacation days.

MY INVESTMENT IN MEDICINE

I have a Bachelor of Arts (B.A.) degree in Biochemistry from a private university. I have a Doctor of Medicine (M.D.) degree and Masters in Business Administration (M.B.A.) degree with specialization in Health Organizational Management from a state-funded school. I am board certified in four medical specialties including Internal Medicine, Cardiovascular Disease, Interventional Cardiology, and Nuclear Cardiology. All of the above represent my 15-year investment in Medicine, for which I still owe approximately $140,000 in student loans.

Trust me, I've done the math many times. According to the Princeton Review, at the time that I'm writing this, the average starting salary for an individual from my undergraduate institution with an M.B.A. is $101,000 per year. Now, let's assume that I never get a raise from my first business job, and I maintain that salary throughout each of the additional years required for medical school, internship, residency, fellowship, and subspecialty fellowship training. Include the time value of money with an 8% rate of annual return. Now, take my current $300,000 annual salary in medicine, subtract the lost revenue from just two weeks of vacation per year in case I finally start taking some, and subtract my debt accumulated from medical school. Add back the low hourly rate that I was paid during the later years of medical training, and include the same 8% rate of annual return mentioned above. All told, it will be 22 years after college, at age 45 years old, when I will finally catch up to myself. This would be the moment when I financially surpass my alter ego with his $101,000 salary, who sadly was never able to receive a promotion within the business world. Without a doubt, I'm not playing this game for the money. In fact, if you'd waive my debt, feed my family, financially provide for my children's education, eliminate the pointless documentation forced upon me for billing in medicine, guarantee I'd never again have to convince a less-informed insurance company what testing or therapy my patient needs, and support the income of my employees who are like a family to me, I'd do the physician part for free.

THE MYTH ABOUT WHY PHYSICIANS CHOOSE MEDICINE

I had a conversation the other day with my brother-in-law. He's an intelligent, highly motivated self-made business man. He was just sharing with me his perception of medicine and physicians. He told me that he was glad that I was in the family because I am someone whom he trusts and from whom he would seek medical advice. I don't even think he receives care from a physician himself, which is interesting because his own perception originates not from any personal experiences, but rather is based upon someone else telling him how he should think about physicians. He told me that you just can't trust some other physicians because you never know when they are being "paid by Pfizer" (Pfizer is a large pharmaceutical corporation) to prescribe certain drugs. The truth is that no physicians are allowed to be paid by a company to prescribe a particular drug. This is obviously illegal. The irony, however, is that I do receive some money from Pfizer, as I'm a part of their physician speaker's bureau.

Ok, so let's think about this. I'm in the game of Life to try and find some way to scam you, make money, and buy a fancy car. I think about the best way to do this, and here's what I decide upon. I'm going to go to a great college, do the very best that I can with my studies, work hard preparing for my standardized medical school entrance exam, apply to medical school, not get accepted the first time around, work harder an additional year gaining experience in basic science research, re-apply to medical school and get in, spend four years in medical school while also concomitantly taking business school classes, graduate with a joint M.D. and M.B.A. degree, spend one year in internship training, two more years in residency, three more in fellowship, and one additional year in subspecialty fellowship training. I finally get out and get my first real job so that I can now scam you by being a physician. This makes absolutely no sense, yet the world and its target-loving media have convinced you otherwise by finding one bad apple to write about in the *Wall Street Journal*.

Physicians aren't alone in this perception. Attorneys have been accused of chasing ambulances, used car salespersons of rolling back the odometer, and mechanics of fixing one part of the vehicle while intentionally breaking another. There is always going to be a *60 Minutes* special that uncovers someone's wrongdoing, and I'm glad for that. The criminals need to be put behind bars. But, it's time for the actions of these people to just be recognized as actions coming from unethical idiots. I don't know where they even find some of these people, but in no way is this representative of my entire profession.

In medical school, I worked long hours in close quarters with about 60 future physicians. In residency, I did the same with almost 80 entirely different people. In fellowship, that number was about 20 more. Over this same time, I interacted with about 65 staff physicians, and since being in private practice, I've gotten to know an additional 30 doctors well. In all this time, I have come across, at the most, one person of questionable ethics. That's less than 0.25% of my physician interactions, and even that one case may have been more of a personality conflict than anything else. The truth is that if you really knew that you had a greater than 99.5% chance that any random mechanic in town would be honest with your car repairs, wouldn't you feel confident that the industry was fantastic?

Indeed, the main issue with healthcare is not fraudulent physicians' behavior, as statistically this is way off-base. The core of the issue remains the perceived value of healthcare as viewed by the consumer, and admittedly, this value is as hard to convey as it is to measure (more on this later).

My Lifestyle

I live on a beautiful two acre lot in a 3,900 square foot home. Adjacent to the home is a separate 900 square foot structure that is my wife's photography studio. Our home, my wife's studio, and the two acre lot cost $815,000 three years ago. I drive a 2012 Ford F150. My wife drives a 2011 Buick Enclave. We own no additional homes, properties, or vehicles. Our formal dining room remains empty of furniture, which is fitting because *formal* doesn't really apply to our style at this stage in life. Perhaps, one day, the room will house a grand piano, which I would enjoy playing.

My wife and I have two young boys, and when I'm not at work, you will most likely find me with them. My boys enjoy the simple things at this stage, playing on the playground, splashing in the puddles in the yard after it rains, and throwing rocks in the lake behind our house. However, our days of little league sports, music recitals, and a myriad of other after school activities appear to be taking shape more and more with each passing day. The challenge to be a good father is much harder for me right now than being a physician, and I work on this daily. Like essentially all of us, I'm a spiritual being, but religion is also a large part of my world. Church serves as a central foundation for me, and my wife and I look for ways daily to share the blessings in our own lives.

I don't golf. For one, I'm terrible, and two, it would take up too much time right now. I don't have any buddies with whom I go on hunting and fishing trips. I have a few good friends, but my wife is my best friend. I do have a few hobbies of my own. For example, I'm writing this book. I routinely go jogging. I have a few business projects on the side (more to come about this later). I do some internet webpage design. But, in general, I consciously try (albeit unsuccessfully at times) to limit some of these personal hobbies, as they only detract from my main focus to be a husband and father. For those of you in that game, you will know what I mean when I say that work is hard enough by itself.

Regarding my physician practice, I share "call" with three other physicians. That means, on average, one out of every four nights I'm readily available for emergencies in the hospital and to answer any patient phone calls after hours. When I'm on call, I have to make a few minor modifications to my lifestyle. I don't drink alcohol anyway, so that one doesn't apply, but of course I refrain from leaving town. My wife and I will take two vehicles to all events, just in case I need to leave suddenly. I can't be counted on to be the only coach at the little league game that night. My wife will schedule none of her photography shoots on those evenings, unless we have a backup plan in place for someone to watch our boys. Call nights just require little adjustments like that to make sure everything runs smoothly.

The messages that I get from patients while on-call are frequently entertaining. You really have to look at it that way or you will have trouble pulling through some of the nights on occasion. I don't get paid to be on call. It's just a service that I have chosen to provide to my patients. And, if you are one of my patients, please don't think that I don't want you to call me when you need me. That's why I'm on call, to help you in a time of need. I just want you to know that I'm compiling a number of entertaining stories that one day will become another book of mine, and that book will entirely be about these phone calls.

In general, the human race is all over the place, and this is never more apparent than my on-call nights. One person, seriously, once called me to ask if I knew of a heart condition that started with the letter "P." I think she must have been playing a game of Scrabble. Another call came from a person who, for whatever reason, had awoken at 3 a.m. to check his blood pressure, and couldn't get his electronic blood pressure monitor to turn on. Midway through the call, he actually paused his train of thought and said: "Man, it just occurred to me, when do you guys ever sleep?" "Well, Sir," I responded, "I actually was sleeping when you called." You just can't make this stuff up.

More recently, I received a call in the middle of the night from a person complaining of chronic diarrhea for six weeks. This may not be as humorous to you as it was for me. For one, the symptoms had been ongoing for over a month, but the patient had finally just decided that she might want to ask someone about them in the middle of the night. And two, I'm a heart doctor. Chronic diarrhea usually isn't something that you are seeing me for anyway.

Stories like this are really for another book at another time, but they do help provide a quick glimpse into a small part of my lifestyle. I want you to know that I still answered those calls as I try to answer every one, with humility and understanding. For one day, I will inevitably be on the other side of that phone call, and I will graciously hope for a similar response.

CHAPTER 2:

The Physician Workaholic is Dying

"MUSICIANS DON'T RETIRE; THEY STOP WHEN
THERE'S NO MORE MUSIC IN THEM."
—LOUIS ARMSTRONG

I n the midst of one of my 110 hour weeks in
fellowship training, the truth first started becoming
apparent to me. Why it took me that long to realize,
I don't know, but they don't teach you this stuff in
medical school. At the time, I had two post-graduate
degrees and one medical board certification behind my
name and was working for the equivalent of $7.86 per
hour. I still had three years to go before completing my
medical training. I realized at that time that I was
nearing a day when, financially, the tables would turn. I

would soon make a fantastic living and start paying off my accumulated debt. I realized that eventually I would earn a great salary, but to do it, I would always be working tirelessly.

At this time, the bane of unnecessary requirements for physician documentation (more about this in Chapter 4) was taking hold. The billing world had become too complex, mostly because of skyrocketing healthcare costs and an apparent distrust of physician decision-making in medicine. Maybe, at some point in the past, physicians somewhere were all being grossly negligent with healthcare costs. But, I'll tell you emphatically, this was not the case on my watch. The physicians training around me were in it for the right reasons, yet we were all caught in the middle of this brewing storm. In the upcoming years, more and more requirements outside of medicine would be forced upon us. We had already started routinely attending billing courses, legal conferences, and computer seminars. We were now being asked to spend time doing the clerical work previously done by several hospital employees, entering our own data and our patients' orders by learning to navigate software systems that we didn't build, we didn't buy, and we couldn't control.

The admission and discharge process for a patient in the hospital was being simplified, we were told. Things would be easier, more efficient, and fewer errors would occur. But, here's what was really happening. The hospital was purchasing buggy computer software programs, firing about four people that previously had assisted the physician in the patient documentation and order entry process, and placing the work of those four individuals back on the physicians. They were doing all of this by hiring a few more administrators to organize more meetings for the physicians to attend to discuss how the hospital could meet specific quality measures in order to market itself as a standard of excellence (don't worry, an entire chapter devoted to these details awaits you shortly).

Still to this day, no data has consistently confirmed better outcomes with any of these new measures. And, just as you don't need data to remind you to wear a parachute when you jump from a plane, you don't need me to tell you that when you are sick, the best thing for you is for your physician to know absolutely everything possible about your disease process. You don't want your physician investing half of his or her energy on things that ultimately deal nothing with figuring out your illness. For example, I can physically draw your blood, process it myself in the computer system and print labels for the test tube, take it down to the lab, run it in the machine, and then create the report of its findings by typing it in an electronic medical record. I can do these things, but this will help little to improve your outcome. In fact, this will only take away from time that I can devote to you.

Returning back to that day in training several years ago, there was finally no doubt in my mind that only tireless hours of work awaited, and that the evolving system was only going to add to my weariness. I would one day make a great salary, but how long would I be able to keep running on the hamster wheel before I would witness my own collapse. Then, it occurred to me: I should buy a vending machine.

THE VENDING MACHINE METAPHOR

A vending machine, in this case, is really meant to be a metaphor. Although, admittedly, a literal vending machine is not that bad of an idea either. A vending machine sits in the corner, is always plugged in, stocked with items to be sold, and essentially runs by itself. Sure, every now and again, you have to restock it, but the owner usually outsources this task anyway. Yes, a vending machine is truly a metaphor for self-sustaining profitability. The owner of the vending machine makes money whenever an item is purchased, and collections occur without the owner needing to be physically present. A vending machine is the perfect analogy of something that makes you money while you sleep.

Many professions are like vending machines. Think about the banking industry, or the real estate and development business. The overriding theme for all of these is ownership and risk. In banking, you actually have to possess money to loan it, and making loans is a risky endeavor. In real estate, you have to own the building to rent it, and there's risk involved with property purchases and finding good tenants. People at the top of these industries work very hard, but the nature of the industry allows for hard work to be done upfront (for example, loaning money that will be paid off in the long-term, when the borrower sends you a check every month with interest). The check can even arrive while you are sleeping.

The dynamics for most physicians is slightly different. You can exist in a non-ownership model, such as being employed by a large healthcare or hospital system where you do not truly own your practice, patients, or equipment. Or, you can go into private practice like me, where you can elect to invest in an ownership strategy by purchasing equipment and medical supplies, but under most circumstances you still must physically be working to earn an income (for example, most medical office testing requires the physical presence of physician oversight and supervision). In either scenario above, the vending machine model fails to hold up.

THE END IS NEARING

Private practice physicians historically have been workaholics. I don't mean this to have a negative connotation. We just previously have really enjoyed what we are doing. We never even thought about this vending machine metaphor. We didn't have time. Too busy doing what we wanted to be doing. But, that was then, and this is now. It's no longer worth it to most physicians remaining in the front lines of patient care to work their tails off. The days of the physician workaholic are literally dying.

I'm too young to even know what it used to be like, but ask around, and the seasoned doctors will paint the picture crystal clear for you. There was a day when seeing patients was less of a chore. You could see 50 patients in a day with one nurse and without breaking a sweat. Then, you could break for lunch, and see 50 more before going to the hospital to round. Unlike the bankers and the real estate moguls, you never made any money when you were sleeping, but that was mainly because you were never sleeping.

Now, for every one doctor, there is a necessity for about a half dozen or more employees, a complex phone and answering service, a full-time billing office, and an information technology department to manage the computer servers for the buggy electronic medical record that you've been required to purchase. Each hospital at which you have privileges to care for your patients has entirely different systems that rarely integrate with each other. In fact, it seems as if you have different name badges, usernames, and passwords for every day of the week. It is literally like you are back in high school, but this time you are not attending classes at just one school. No, you are at many schools, the one in your neighborhood, the rival one across town, and some third place in a different zip code. And, the school supply list is entirely different at each place. One hospital has a vendor contract that requires you to use this type of #2 pencil for your heart catheterization while the other hospital doesn't even have a pencil for you to use at all. Your entire day, both in the clinic and at the hospital, is spent meandering through operational systems too cumbersome, too tiring, and frankly just too annoying to work within.

This is why you are getting out.

THE EXIT STRATEGY

The easiest way out is to move gracefully into a healthcare administrative role. For one, you've seen this gig from the outside for a while now. You've seen what they do: carry their cup of coffee from meeting to meeting. You can do this. You admit that it won't improve your job satisfaction, but you will get paid a fair salary, and you can quit taking overnight call at the hospital. Besides, it will be a new game to play trying to get to the top of that world, and this will entertain you for a bit.

Your second option is to become an employed physician within a large healthcare system. Here you will have safety in numbers. You will have lots of other doctors to herd around with and this means that you will have some camaraderie. Most all of these employment situations have an established productivity model, so you can still crank out the work if you want to. But, there is something that you should know. The statistics actually say that you won't do this. You will giddy up for several years, but ultimately you'll realize that the incentives that they are giving you are not worth the extra work. Why? Because every corporate system has a legal structure designed around taking advantage of cheap labor. No, the statistics say that you'll eventually start to look for ways to supplement your income with non-clinical (more administrative) duties. Indeed, the days of the physician workaholic in this model have long sense passed.

MY FIRST VENDING MACHINE

Midway through my fellowship training in cardiovascular disease, my program director asked me if it were possible to electronically track the number of electrocardiograms (ECGs) that my colleagues and I read every day. An ECG, for those of you who don't know, is a bunch of squiggly lines on a piece of paper that account for your heart's electrical activity. It kind of looks like the output generated by one of those lie detector tests, with a marked fluctuation in scribble surrounding each heartbeat.

As a part of your training in medicine, especially in the field of cardiology, you spend a lot of time learning how to understand and read these ECGs. And, you must read a whole bunch of these things to become proficient, like thousands and thousands, because this is the technology that enables you to rapidly detect heart attacks or other heart arrhythmias that can be life-threatening to your patients. I was already reading thousands of these ECGs each year in my training. I might read one that was just performed on my patient at the bedside, place my comments at the top of the printed out page, and put this paper copy in the chart. Then, I'd move on to the next patient. But, nobody was documenting what I was doing. There was no proof of how many that I was reading, because no logical recording system was in place. My program director knew about my knowledge in computers and webpage design and wondered if a solution were possible.

I saw potential in this project, but for a different reason. Like all medical trainees, I ultimately would be taking self-assessment Board Exams. On these Board Exams, especially the ones for cardiology, I would have to master a number of these ECGs in order to pass the test. The ECG questions on this board exam would use a unique score sheet with nearly 100 different diagnoses. That's like a multiple choice test having not just letters A through Z, but A through Z in 4 different columns, which as you might imagine, can make things very challenging. This test is something that you would definitely need to prepare for accordingly.

At the time of my training, however, there was essentially only one good book available to help you study for this Board Exam. Moreover, this exam had just recently transitioned to an all-computer-based format. Computer exams have different dynamics such as clicking a mouse and toggling back-and-forth between virtual windows on the screen, which makes preparing for it with a hardcopy book less optimal anyway. Instead, imagine a web-based study guide where you could learn and read these ECGs on a computer in an identical format to the Board Exam, using a similar score sheet.

Out of this idea, I developed ECGsource.com, the largest online resource for electrocardiograms and related Board Exam imaging preparation.

ECGSOURCE.COM

I didn't know that I was developing a small vending machine at that time, but I was. I outsourced almost nothing. I collected all of the content myself, hard-coded the website myself, integrated it for online subscription payment processing myself, and launched it with a marketing budget of zero. At about the same time, the smartphone mobile application industry was exploding, so I figured why not build an iPhone Operating System (iOS) supplemental application to go along with the website.

I could have looked for a real iOS developer to help me out, but I didn't. I have some knowledge of web-based programming, but no formal training in programming languages like C++ or Objective-C, which are typically what developer kits for these type of systems are based upon. But, this is a unique time in history when you can essentially build a rocket to the moon by watching a YouTube video, so why not give it a try yourself.

First, came the mobile application, ECGsource, for the iPhone OS. Then, came a second mobile application, CathSource, a medical reference for cardiac catheterization and angiography, and finally, a third, EchoSource, an application devoted to the field of echocardiography. Basically, all of these applications contain content not only helpful for a beginner learning about these specialties in medicine, but useful as a pocket reference for practicing clinicians. I would eventually create versions of these mobile applications available for the Android Operation System as well.

For the record, my Apps are nothing like Angry Birds. (If you are lost in this world of mobile technology, Angry Birds is a video game franchise that has become arguably one of the greatest mobile application success stories of all time, achieving more than two billion downloads across all platforms and this number is constantly growing.) The first day my ECGsource App was available, about a dozen downloads occurred worldwide. With my marketing budget of zero, I'm not really sure how anyone even found it in the App store, but they did. The wild thing was that the next day, a few more people downloaded it, and then a few more. In fact, to the best of my knowledge, nearly every day since then over the last few years, at least one person somewhere has found one of my Apps to download. I recall that I even had one lucky day where my Apps were downloaded 351 times, which still remains my all-time daily record.

Indeed, on this day, I finally made money while I was sleeping.

THE NEXT 10 YEARS

Over the next 10 years, unless changes occur within our healthcare system, the physician workaholic will become like an enshrined statue at the museum, a lasting memory of a prior age. In fact, physicians in their middle-to-late twilight years have already been checking out in the express line for some time. If you are like me and consider yourself relatively young at heart in this poker game of medicine, you may be willing to hold your hand of cards for another decade on the off chance that a surprising "river card" will be dealt that changes healthcare's anticipated dreary outcome. You may take the path less traveled and fight to survive as a private practitioner, or you may elect to implement one of the exit strategies discussed above.

The problem with you getting out is that you are really good at what you do, and the system is going to suffer from your exit. The quality of care will go down, along with access to it. But it's just no longer worth it to sustain yourself as a workaholic in this environment. If someone could change a few things with the system you'd consider coming back. Or, if your vending machine takes off, you'd do the physician thing on your own terms for free, because you really love taking care of patients. It's just the other things that bring you down. Healthcare quality measures, which cost millions of dollars to implement, mean essentially nothing for the patients because they're merely administrative check boxes. Absurd medical documentation requirements abound that have no business being a part of any business. The process for maintaining your own physician licensure and board certification is dreadful, and on top of that, you are wasting more and more time arguing with insurance companies on behalf of your patients.

You'll learn more about all of these things in the chapters to come, but this is precisely why the physician workaholic is dying. All that's left is folks carrying their coffee from meeting to meeting. If these people with their caffeinated beverages would just listen to you fighting from the front lines of patient care, they could help you fix this debacle.

CHAPTER 3:

The Futility of Most Healthcare Quality Measures

"IF THE BLIND LEAD THE BLIND, BOTH
SHALL FALL INTO THE DITCH."
—MATTHEW 15:14

What you are about to read is not popular. My comments will be deemed controversial by most major medical societies, but I'm not writing this book to make friends. I'm writing this because I believe what I'm saying is right, and I believe that you deserve more than half the story when it comes to understanding healthcare quality. I want to help solve our problems, and the first step is to understand the areas where we've got it all wrong. Mainly, if you are ever going to find value again in medicine, you've got to know who can be counted on to be your Consumer Report, and I promise you that it's not going to be who you think.

First, I want to define *quality measures* in healthcare, because I'm fairly confident that if you haven't been exposed to this type of thing already, you soon will be. In part due to the signing into law of the Patient Protection and Affordable Care Act (ACA) in 2010, quality measures are becoming increasingly linked to both hospitals and physicians. I will discuss more about the ACA in later chapters, but quality measures, in general, simply entail how well something is being done compared to an established standard. In medicine, this might be how quickly a hospital is able to render care to you in an emergency situation such as a heart attack, or how adequately your doctor is treating your diabetes.

As a kid growing up in the 1980s, I closely followed Wade Boggs, who at the time was a third baseman for the Boston Red Sox. Every morning I enjoyed opening the sports page of our local newspaper and turning to the Major League Baseball statistics section. I usually was most interested in tracking the batting averages of the best hitters in the league. If baseball is not your pastime, a batting average is the percentage of time a baseball hitter reaches base successfully with a hit. A batting average is essentially one quality measure in baseball, and a really good hitter is able to consistently get more than 3 hits for every 10 at bats, or maintain a batting average greater than .300.

Boggs is now in the Baseball Hall of Fame, having recorded more than 3,000 hits in his 18-year career. In the 1980s, he was just beginning his career, but he would win five American League batting titles before the decade was complete. A batting title means that he had the very best batting average in his league during those years. In fact, in the six seasons spanning 1983 to 1988, he had the highest batting average in all of Major League Baseball on four occasions, including his career best average of .368 in 1985.

A batting average, in general, is very straightforward to calculate. You divide your number of hits by your official number of at bats. There are only a few subtleties with its calculation. For example, you do not get credit for a hit when someone on the other team makes an error (or mistake) allowing you to get on base. Special situations termed walks and sacrifice plays, both of which are easily recognizable and well-defined in the baseball rule book, neither count for you as hits nor against you as at bats when calculating your batting average. In almost all instances, however, for any fan watching the game, it is extremely straightforward to figure out when a player gets a hit. If there is any question, an official scorekeeper will make the final decision. In fact, in his entire career, Wade Boggs never once got to decide if he got a hit. He was never involved with this official process of calculating his batting average. All he had to do was go up to the plate and bat.

On the surface, quality measures in healthcare seem to make a lot of sense. You can see how they might be viewed as like batting averages for hospitals and physicians. In fact, let's pay physicians and hospitals bonuses for having high batting averages, while penalizing them for low ones. Statistics like this surely can help us determine who deserves to be on a medicine All-Star Team, right? As it turns out, comparing batting averages works exceptionally well in baseball, a game with a fairly level playing field and standardized rules. Every game is played with the same-sized ball, the same distance from the pitching mound to the hitter, and the same number of bases. Unfortunately, there is one ginormous problem with how this relates to healthcare; healthcare is absolutely nothing like baseball.

HEMOGLOBIN A1C AS A QUALITY MEASURE

Hemoglobin A1c (HbA1c) is a common blood test used to evaluate for the presence of diabetes and to monitor blood sugar control in your body. Hemoglobin is a molecule inside your red blood cells responsible for carrying oxygen to all your organs. Think of HbA1c as being the percentage of your hemoglobin bound to sugar molecules. The greater the number of sugar molecules floating in your blood stream, the higher your HbA1c will be. In fact, since hemoglobin-containing red blood cells have a lifespan of only a few months, your HbA1c level provides a very good estimate of your body's average blood sugar over the preceding three months.

High sugar levels impair appropriate functioning of your organs, which is why diabetes can be such a debilitating disease. Think of what happens when you spill a sugar-containing soft drink on the floor and don't clean it up. Once the floor dries, it will become very sticky because of the sugar. This is essentially what happens on the inside of your cells when you have uncontrolled diabetes. All the enzymes that need to constantly interact with each other in order to create useful chemical reactions become "gummed up" by all the sugar molecules. Your entire cellular factory will ultimately shut down if your sugar levels cannot be controlled. This is why it is important for your doctor to help you keep your HbA1c level as low as possible.

In fact, why not make HbA1c levels a healthcare quality measure? This should be very straightforward. For example, if your doctor is better than anyone else at treating diabetes, your doctor's patients will surely have the lowest HbA1c levels. If your physician really cares about you and knows what he or she is doing, your physician will spend an incessant amount of time working with you until your HbA1c level is controlled. Doctors' batting averages for HbA1c can then be used to compare one doctor to another, and the world will suddenly become a better place. I just hope that if you really believe that last statement, you'll read this chapter twice.

To illustrate, Dr. X and Dr. Y both treat patients with diabetes. As a part of new government-driven processes supposedly assessing quality in healthcare, both doctors submit data regarding HbA1c levels of their diabetic patients for review. A good HbA1c level is less than 6.5%, whereas a bad one is above 9%. Dr. X and Dr. Y have thousands of patients, including many at either end of the spectrum. However, Dr. X has a much higher percentage of patients with suboptimal HbA1c levels over 9%. In fact, 42% of Dr. X's patients have HbA1c levels above this cutoff value. Dr. Y's patients fare much better, with only 14% having this high of HbA1c levels.

If this were baseball, Dr. Y would be the superior player hands down. Why? Because Dr. Y keeps his patients' blood sugar levels the lowest, and this means improved quality and lower cost for the healthcare system. Fewer of his patients will go on to develop complications of diabetes such as kidney failure, and less of his folks will require expensive medical therapies such as dialysis. If you had diabetes, surely you'd rather be cared for by Dr. Y. For crying out-loud, Dr. Y's batting average is three times better!

But before you schedule your appointment with Dr. Y, let me tell you a few more things about these two physicians. Dr. X practices medicine in an inner-city academic hospital and is a specialist in diabetes management. She actually trained a few additional years in order to manage the most challenging patients and has over 100 publications in her area of expertise. Smart physicians who can't get their patients' diabetes under control actually send their patients to see Dr. X as a last hope. Dr. X's patients often don't have enough money to afford the best medicines, they tend to be less educated about disease processes, and they have weaker community support systems.

Dr. Y practices in an affluent suburb. He is a great doctor, too, but hasn't trained as many years as Dr. X. His patients almost always have good insurance and can afford the best medications. They are very well-educated with strong support systems with typically unlimited access to exercise facilities, personal trainers, and dietary counselors. Dr. Y works very hard to help his patients, but it makes absolutely no sense to compare his batting average to Dr. X. The two physicians aren't really even playing the same game. Dr. X sees sicker patients with fewer resources. Her batting average on a day-to-day basis is meaningless. Her peers know that her reputation for quality in diabetes management is unsurpassed, which is why they send their most challenging patients to see her. Dr. X is actually the one whom you should be fighting to see.

MEDICINE IS STILL AN ART FORM

I'd like to put something in perspective for you. I mean absolutely no disrespect to the scientific minds that have played such a crucial role in the development of Western medicine over the years, but I want you to know that medicine is much less of a perfect science than you really think that it is. You'll learn more about the imperfections of clinical studies later in this book, but it's important that you realize a little bit about this concept now. In fact, it's not just an uneven physician playing field that makes a majority of quality measures in medicine meaningless, it's the fact that assessing quality is still as subjective as it gets.

In the mid-1980s, about the same time that I was intently following Wade Boggs and his batting average, a landmark clinical trial was performed that would forever change our approach in treating patients with heart attacks. The trial was called the Second International Study of Infarct Survival[1] but is better known in the cardiology community as ISIS-2. ISIS-2 would ultimately provide a number of helpful conclusions, but one of these is that Aspirin appeared to be useful when given to individuals in the setting of a heart attack.

In this study, a group of patients having heart attacks were allocated oral Aspirin and compared to others receiving a Placebo tablet (also known as a "sham" therapy). Either therapy was administered on a daily basis, and after 35 days of treatment, the group of people receiving Aspirin died less frequently. Specifically, the Aspirin group had an absolute 2.4% risk reduction in death from vascular causes (basically death from a heart attack or stroke). But, don't get too focused on the numbers yet. This study is telling you that Aspirin works, and I'm glad that it does, because I'm a cardiologist and I want to help my patients. But, this chapter is about more than what meets the eye, so let's look deeper together at how great of a benefit Aspirin really seems to be providing us when we are having a heart attack.

I already told you that overall it was better for you to have been in the Aspirin group. But, do you know that 9.4% of the people receiving Aspirin still died a vascular death by five weeks' time? This means that, unfortunately, Aspirin wasn't able to save those individuals. For this group of people, Aspirin provided no survival value. Moreover, do you know that 88.2% of the patients who never even received Aspirin were still alive at 35 days? That means that nearly 9 out of 10 people were going to survive anyway, regardless of what we did, without the help or need for Aspirin.

One vocabulary word that often is mentioned when evaluating data in clinical trials is something known as *number needed to treat*. This just means how many people that you would have to treat with a study medication before you could definitively prove that you prevented one bad thing. The lower that this number is, the more beneficial a therapy has been proven to be. In the ISIS-2 trial, the number of people needed to be treated with Aspirin to prevent one vascular death at five weeks was 42 individuals. This means that the *number needed to treat* was 42. In the business of clinical trials, this is actually a fairly good (meaning low) *number needed to treat* value. Yet, this can really be interpreted in two different ways. The first way, is what I've already told you, that Aspirin worked. But, the second way is that you had to give Aspirin to 42 people before it finally helped one of them. Statistically speaking, for 41 out of the 42 people taking Aspirin, the medicine provided absolutely no survival benefit.

So, in the setting of a heart attack, Aspirin was found to be superior compared to doing nothing, but Aspirin didn't win by a landslide. It won by a photo finish. And, trust me, Aspirin's *number needed to treat* is better than most drugs approved out there for different types of indications. In fact, Aspirin is viewed as such a "quality" medication for you to take when having a heart attack, that using it is one of those hospital quality measures that Medicare looks at when deciding if it's going to adjust its payments to a hospital. For this very reason, hospitals literally hire full-time employees to be administrators for quality measures. These people don't go around and provide additional care for patients who've had heart attacks, although to me this would actually seem to improve quality. Instead, they just fill out a bunch of paperwork documenting that Aspirin has been given, since documenting the use of Aspirin clearly provides a landslide of value. Whom are we kidding? Actually taking the Aspirin doesn't even provide a landslide of value.

The point that I am making here is that we are spending *tons* of resources and funds trying to administrate healthcare quality measures that don't add much quality. All this extraneous stuff isn't needed. In fact, do you know what else has been proven to save your life when you are having a heart attack? Believe it or not, it's actually your physician. You probably forgot about that person, as the doctor can be hard to find these days amongst all the administrators and documenters. Regardless, when having a heart attack, just receiving treatment from a heart specialist (for example, a cardiologist), instead of a primary care physician, lowers your in-hospital death rate by 17%. Being cared for by a physician who manages a high volume of heart attack patients every year, basically a doctor who has seen this type of thing before, reduces your mortality by 11%.[2] All you need when you are really sick is the best-trained doctor available and quality will take care of itself. You don't need a bunch of folks in meetings coming up with meaningless metrics and pseudo-certifications. We've already been doing that for several years now, and I'm about to show you what we've created.

CHEST PAIN CENTER ACCREDITATION

I got a junk email today that I have to tell you about. I usually get one like this every other week or at least an equivalent letter once per month in the mail. I suspect that you get these from time to time yourself. The email message that I received today told me that I had won an award. Specifically, I was selected for a best of City honor. Evidently, I was chosen because I've used various marketing methods to grow a small business in spite of difficult economic times. I wasn't even sure what they were talking about, so I went to the organization's website just for fun. This organization is actually a real one, or at least they appear to be. They claim to be looking for companies in my town that exemplify the best in small business, and they are recognizing me for implementing programs that generate competitive advantages and long-term value. On the main page of their website, they provide me a direct link to enter my business number and claim my award. They will send me a blue crystal plaque to display on my desk for all to see. They will distribute a press release to the local newspaper explaining my award. In fact, they make it clear that if I use this award effectively, it can become another sales tool to aid in the growth of my business. Who knows, they may actually even be right. Probably someone who visits me in my office will really think that this award means something. And, all this organization needs for me to do is PAY THEM FOR THE COST OF MY OWN AWARD!

You and I laugh at this ridiculous junk email and call it a scam. But, this scenario is nearly identical to many of the certifications your hospital is either currently getting or has already obtained. I'll tell you about one such award that I know plenty about because it deals with my area of expertise. My colleagues and I once did all the work for our hospital to get it. In fact, the next time that you see a hospital billboard, see if you can find a seal of approval on it. The one that I'm talking about is called: "Chest Pain Center Accreditation."

Heart attack remains the number cause of death in our society today. I've essentially devoted my professional life to educate, diagnosis, prevent, and treat people with heart disease. I'm on the front lines taking care of these patients, but I'm not the only one who has gotten involved with the process. The Society of Cardiovascular Patient Care (SCPC) is an organization who mentions on its website that it's committed to eliminating heart disease by improving hospital protocols through Accreditation processes. The SCPC originated out of the concept to create what is termed a Chest Pain Center at every hospital. Chest pain is a common presenting symptom for individuals coming into the emergency department, and you need a streamlined process to manage these people effectively. The SCPC was established not only on the premise of rapidly treating individuals with heart attacks in these Chest Pain Centers, but also with the intent of informing the community at large about Early Heart Attack Care (EHAC).

I actually like all of SCPC's idealistic goals, but their Accreditation processes have become another prime example of a third-party being unsuccessful at creating quality in healthcare. According to SCPC's own website, EHAC is an educational process founded on "common sense measures." The rather humorous thing is that I could not have summarized SCPC's entire operation any better myself. Literally, they have evolved from those idealistic goals into an organization which essentially gives out awards for Common Sense that YOU MUST PAY FOR YOURSELF.

You can't make this stuff up. You want your hospital to be Accredited in Common Sense? Pay the SCPC $22,000 and they'll explain what you need to do to claim your award. That's the actual cost this year for your hospital to receive Chest Pain Center Accreditation. Once you pay that off, feel free to write them another check to have your hospital also Accredited in Atrial Fibrillation and Heart Failure. Those disease processes I treat every day and they are the newest certifications offered by SCPC.

What's involved with claiming your award from SCPC other than paying your funds? Well, you get to pay for some people to go to a workshop. To be honest, the SCPC actually wants you to hire a full-time employee just to oversee this process of obtaining your award. That's another expense. Anyway, you send this full-time Chest Pain Center person from your hospital to a workshop. Then, you receive a binder (this is how it used to be, but now almost everything is submitted online) that you go through page by page, checking off lists of things that any hospital wanting to attract market share in cardiac care is already doing. For example, you should have signage on your property that appropriately helps ambulances find your emergency department. Take a picture and submit it as proof. Make a copy of some educational material that you are providing your heart attack patients. By the way, this printed material has never been shown to affect patient outcomes, but since you are doing it anyway, this is an easy box to check to meet some of SCPC's patient education requirements. Your full-time Chest Pain Center Coordinator then needs to convince one of your hospital's physicians to be the Medical Director of the Chest Pain Center. Usually, this will end up being a physician who is already employed by your hospital, because everyone else will be less motivated to participate in another hospital bureaucratic experiment.

I have to be honest with you. When I was directly involved with this affair for one of my hospitals, there was actually ONE new thing that we started doing that we weren't doing prior to going through this Accreditation process. We began taking FORMAL ATTENDANCE at our monthly Heart Attack meeting.

We had never done that before. We just had never written down everyone's name who was in attendance at that hospital committee meeting. We started doing that, and once SCPC received our money, we claimed our Chest Pain Center Accreditation award.

You actually get to keep your Accreditation for three years. After that, you pay more money to do it all again. But don't worry, they'll add a few more things for you the next time. It's like reading the next edition of a textbook. Some of the sentences might be different. For Chest Pain Center Accreditation, the current version is called CPC v5. I guess that is like the fifth reiteration. Previously, they referred to them as cycles. But, one thing is certain: they'll make sure to tell you that their newest generation of check boxes will add more quality to your hospital.

Now, I don't want you to think that these people involved with SCPC are bad people. They're not. In fact, they actually believe that what they are doing is good. But, we just don't need third parties mooching off the system offering certifications in common sense. You, the patient, are indirectly paying for this nonsense. Every time that you go to the hospital, and they send you a bill, whether you pay it or your insurance pays it, some of that revenue generated by the hospital is going toward paying for meaningless Accreditations. The moochers want you to believe that all of this is necessary for you to receive quality care, but high-quality low-cost care just isn't finding its way through all of the added layers of complexity.

The amazing thing is that, to date, SCPC has had over 1,000 hospitals purchase an Accreditation award from them. And, I'm sure that number will continue to grow, especially since they keep adding more Accreditations for other disease processes. Feel free to do the math. They are generating a lot of revenue for a not-for-profit organization. How in the world are they getting all these hospital administrators to buy into their awards scheme? Easy. They somehow have everyone convinced that Medicare is about to stop making payments to any hospital treating chest pain that is not Accredited by SCPC. I'm telling you that was the rumor five years ago, and it's still the rumor today. Maybe they know something we don't know. But, seriously, this hasn't ever happened. Moreover, I'm unaware of anything like this coming down the pipeline, yet hospitals keep purchasing these seals of approval for their billboards. Unbelievable.

THE JOINT COMMISSION

SCPC is far from being the only third-party from which your hospital can purchase a medal of honor. There are a myriad of groups like these out there, with the biggest player probably being an organization known as The Joint Commission (TJC). TJC has gone by several different names over the years including the Joint Commission on Accreditation of Hospitals (JCAH) and the Joint Commission on Accreditation of Healthcare Organizations (JCAHO), but they've been known as TJC since 2007.

It would take an entire separate book to outline everything that I really want to tell you about TJC, but it's important that we at least scratch the surface of this organization now. Government-funded Medicare/Medicaid is the single largest health insurer in the United States. In order for healthcare facilities to participate in its programs, which means getting paid for rendering care to Medicare and Medicaid patients, these facilities must meet the Centers for Medicare and Medicaid Services (CMS) Conditions of Participation (CoPs). Think of CoPs as being certain standards that your hospital must meet in order to be worthy of CMS funds. As a hospital, you typically have several options for demonstrating that you meet these standards. You can be evaluated by CMS directly, by a State agency, or by an Accreditation agency that CMS has authorized. Regarding the last option, CMS has granted TJC something known as a "deemed status," which really just means that if TJC thinks your hospital's standards are okay, CMS will agree and therefore pay you for services rendered to its Medicare and Medicaid patients. TJC used to have a monopoly in this third-party CMS Accreditation world. Thankfully, however, this is not the case anymore, but the majority of hospitals in this country still use TJC to satisfy the standards set forth by CMS.

TJC, like SCPC, charges hospitals tens-of-thousands of dollars to obtain Accreditation. There have been numerous critics of TJC over the years regarding its success, or rather lack thereof, at actually improving the quality of healthcare facilities. But, I'm not here to bash TJC. Their job, as they are trying to do it, is literally impossible, mainly because their methodology is designed to fail. Quality isn't derived merely from strong-arming hospitals into creating excessive policies and procedures that TJC can inspect to make sure that they are in place. In fact, too much administration of check boxes actually causes you to lose focus on what you are trying to do in the first place, which is to enable physicians, nurses, therapists, technicians, and the other medical personnel teams to actually take care of patients. We've already learned this lesson about quality from the decades long case-study better known as the Veteran's Administration (VA) Healthcare System, which I'll brief you on later in the book. No, TJC has been working really hard in the name of quality. They've expanded immensely upon the standards set forth by CMS, but in all the wrong ways. I have no qualms with their efforts, but their philosophy on what drives quality in healthcare is terribly flawed.

In 2013, according to the United States Census Bureau, for every 100 people aged 25 years or older in America, 88 had managed to graduate from high school.

Almost 32 of these 100 individuals succeeded in obtaining at least a Bachelor's Degree in College, and about eight people had obtained a Master's Degree. Roughly 1% of these 100 individuals had successfully obtained a professional degree such as law or medicine. In fact, according to the *2013 State Physician Workforce Data Book* put out by the Association of American Medical Colleges, physicians represent 0.26%, or one-fourth of 1%, of the United States population. The rigorous medical education process by itself selects out a limited few to be Accredited as physicians.

Let's contrast that to TJC, whose goal in accrediting organizations is to inspire healthcare facilities to excel at providing safe and effective care of the highest quality and value. TJC historically has accredited more than 99% of the hospitals that it inspects. Imagine signing up to take a class where essentially no one fails, and then bragging about yourself when you pass. How does that type of system ignite any drive for quality? Besides having a flawed philosophy on how best to improve value, the main issue that I have with TJC is that nearly everyone who wants to receive their award, pays their money and gets it. In fact, TJC even has a for-profit affiliate, Joint Commission Resources (JCR), that sells TJC's Accreditation manuals and offers pricey consulting services, including "mock" surveys, to help your hospital better prepare for TJC's inspection. Why pay once to get an award when you can pay twice to GUARANTEE that you'll get the award?

In more recent years, TJC has even gotten into the business of issuing more so-called "Advanced Certifications" to centers making "exceptional efforts" to improve outcomes related to certain disease-specific states. Basically, what SCPC is now doing with chest pain, heart failure, and atrial fibrillation Accreditations, TJC is doing for kidney disease, stroke, lung diseases, end-of-life care, and also heart failure. I wish that I could get excited about all these plaques that you can purchase for your wall, but the true reality—and this is coming from someone on the inside of the circus—is that all of these certifications are relatively meaningless.

I once worked at a hospital that held TJC's Certificate of Distinction for being a Primary Stroke Center. This just means that this facility was supposedly the place in the community that you would want to go to if you had experienced the unfortunate circumstance of having had a stroke. A stroke is a condition where you suddenly lose brain function, typically in a localized area, perhaps leading to strength or sensation loss in your extremity or troubles with your speech. Strokes can be caused from blood clots developing inside the arteries of your brain, or even from bleeding itself within the brain. The facility that I worked at was proud of this TJC distinction and marketed this certification every way that it could. In fact, you could call this facility on the phone, and if you had to be placed on hold for any reason, an automated speaker would come on the line and tell you all about how this center was a Primary Stroke Center.

One day, I was caring for a patient who suffered a stroke at this hospital. I did what is typical in a situation where the disease process involves the brain, and I consulted a brain doctor, or neurologist, to help me with the case. What ensued is as bizarre as anything that I've been a part of in medicine. This Primary Stroke Center that I worked at did not even have a neurologist available on-site that day to see my patient. For those of you familiar with George Lucas's *Star Wars* films, you'll understand my next analogy well. The nurse literally rolled in this R2-D2 - like robotic device with a camera on top so that my patient could visit with a neurologist by a satellite somewhere. Say what? You can't even make this stuff up, and it even gets better. As it turned out, the R2-D2 device didn't even work. The neurologist had to speak to my patient by phone.

For those of you not in medicine, you should know that a neurologist's greatest asset is often his or her ability to perform an incredibly thorough physical exam. This typically involves testing nerves throughout the body with pins, reflex hammers, and tuning forks, and evaluating a patient's strength through resistance maneuvers. Now, try doing all of that over the phone. I'll give you the fact that the neurologist on the phone that day would at least have been able to assess whether my patient could hear him, but the remainder of the neurological assessment was obviously unbelievably limited. And, this my friends, was at one of TJC's distinguished centers for stroke. When it was needed, there was no ability for a specialist to perform an on-site neurological exam, but those administrators had clearly spent thousands of dollars checking off all the right boxes to get a stroke certificate. Too bad this advanced certification was meaningless for my patient.

THE PHYSICIAN QUALITY REPORTING SYSTEM

Starting in 2015, as specified by the ACA, a physician's reimbursement from Medicare will become reduced by 1.5% if that physician did not participate in CMS's Physician Quality Reporting System (PQRS) for the 2013 calendar year. The PQRS currently just involves physicians submitting their own quality metrics, such as data regarding their patient's HbA1c levels, to CMS for review. If the physician elects not to participate by submitting at least nine variables in 2014, a 2% penalty will be levied on the physician in 2016. Think of PQRS as being CMS's attempt to provide incentives to physicians to improve quality in healthcare. I love the concept, but as you've already learned, trying to measure quality in medicine with batting averages doesn't work very well. Even if there was one quality measure that really meant something to track, you'd only be doing any good if the data used to compute that quality measure could be counted on to be truly accurate. Hence, I present to you the other major obstacle for quality assessment in healthcare, overcoming poor or inaccurate data collection.

I have an electronic medical record (EMR) in my office. This ultimately costs me tens-of-thousands of dollars every year to maintain and just means that I use a computer system to document patient visits, report office testing, and manage patient medications. I'm required to use entirely different EMRs at each of the two hospitals where I see patients currently. I'm in favor of using EMR systems; in fact, as you've already learned about me, computer programming is one of my business hobbies. But, just know that none of these three EMRs interacts with each other, all are very buggy, and technical support is rarely helpful at fixing any of the problems that physicians know exist. In fact, the entire EMR situation in medicine right now is a microcosm of our entire healthcare system. Physicians and medical providers are no longer central to patient care. Systems aren't built around these groups of frontline workers in an effort to enable them. Instead, the system itself has become the centerpiece. Providers have become interchangeable pawns, almost like pieces of gum being stuck to a rolling wheel, and you wonder why quality isn't getting any better. You don't need a good piano teacher anymore. You just need an average sounding piano and your students will somehow learn to play better on their own.

On an annual basis, I submit to CMS the PQRS data collected from my EMR. At this time, I still remain a participant in this PQRS debacle, but as you are about to see, if I lived entirely by principle, I would have thrown in the towel long ago due to its inherent futility. Regardless, when I submit my PQRS data, I'm required to submit the precise numbers outputted by my EMR, whether those numbers are really correct or not. I'll give you some rather humorous examples.

For the 2012 calendar year, my EMR calculated that 82% of my patients with heart disease were given medications to help treat their cholesterol. CMS evidently feels this is an important quality measure, and I don't entirely disagree. Certain cholesterol medications do improve outcomes in patients with heart disease. One interesting thing with this metric, however, is that CMS counts **all** cholesterol medications the same. What if I prescribe you a medicine known as a *bile acid sequestrant,* which happens to be a cholesterol medication, but for reasons not entirely clear, has never been shown to actually lower your risk of a heart attack? By doing this, I would look favorable in the eyes of this metric, while perhaps not doing anything at all of quality for your heart disease. Regarding my 82% success rate, that number actually doesn't make me out to be too bad of a doctor. I'm sure that some appropriate reasons existed that weren't picked up by my EMR that might explain why the other 18% weren't taking these medications. Perhaps, even some of my patients had refused or couldn't afford them. But, the most humorous thing to me is that my 82% metric was calculated from a denominator of 39 patients. That's right. My EMR determined that I only saw 39 patients for the entire year who actually had heart disease. I'm a heart doctor. My entire clinic is full of these people. I see 39 people with heart disease every week. But, I only can submit what my EMR spits out, so that's the data that CMS has on me. I'm sure they are busy studying that data and making conclusions about me. Good or bad, those conclusions will be worthless, because the data that led to them was flawed.

This last year, I supposedly saw 557 patients who were eligible for me to ask them about tobacco use. My EMR determined that I "assessed" absolutely NONE of them, meaning that I never even asked one person for the entire year if they smoked cigarettes. Of the zero people that I asked, I obviously counseled zero regarding tobacco cessation, which gave me a 0% success rate for tobacco assessment and intervention. I guess that I must have tied for last in this category for heart doctors in America, because I'm not aware that you can submit negative numbers. The irony is that this is actually something that I do very well. In fact, CMS even paid me last year for performing tobacco cessation. Believe it or not, because of its importance for overall health, CMS will pay a doctor an additional few dollars for an office visit, not to exceed two visits per patient per year, in which the doctor performs a few minutes of tobacco cessation counseling. I submitted numerous claims to CMS regarding the time that I spent with tobacco cessation counseling. These claims were submitted through my EMR to CMS, and CMS appropriately paid me, yet for whatever reason, my EMR still recorded me as being 0% in this PQRS category.

Now, you might think that the problem is my EMR. Or, maybe you think that I don't know how to use my EMR properly. And, perhaps at some level you might be correct. You think that my EMR is only as good as the information that I put in it. But, I want you to know this: I pay for multiple employees to attend conferences each year for them to learn how to input information appropriately on my behalf into my EMR. Moreover, as you learned in the first few chapters, I am a closet computer programmer. I've hard-coded on my spare time three different iPhone applications and three more for the Android mobile platform. I develop web pages by being self-taught on HTML, JavaScript, Flash, and PHP programing languages. I manage my own server. If I happen to also be a physician and still can't figure this thing out, they should literally throw the system away.

Now, all things considered, don't you worry about me. On top of my other commitments, notwithstanding my attempt to be the best physician to my patients that I can be, I became so frustrated after two consecutive years with the ridiculous 0% number, that I figured out the glitch myself in my EMR. I've now built my own template, as recommended by my EMR vendor, and I've been implementing that new template for this year. Now when I perform tobacco cessation counseling, I make certain to check five additional boxes per patient on the EMR screen. This year is not complete yet, but I ran my PQRS numbers the other day and I'm literally 100% in this category. In fact, as it turns out, my EMR is not even tabulating failed tobacco assessments any more. Unbelievable. It's like my EMR's new template only counts shots when I make the basket, which makes absolutely no sense. I will literally go from 0% to 100% in a single year for this metric, doing precisely the same quality of job that I've always done, and frankly, neither number is even right.

I could literally go on and on about physician quality measures and the widespread challenges resulting from poor data entry. Moreover, don't think for a second that this is limited to only government-developed CMS measures. This exists throughout the entire healthcare industry, just due to the nature of medical complexity. One of my former colleagues, who is also a Board Certified Interventional Cardiologist, just received feedback on the data being submitted on his behalf to the National Cardiovascular Data Registry (NCDR). This NCDR was developed by the American College of Cardiology, a not-for-profit medical society of which I'm an active member. The NCDR encompasses six hospital-based registries and one outpatient registry, with the term registry just implying that it's an enormous collection of data regarding both physician procedures and medical care in the specialty of cardiovascular disease. One of NCDR's registries specifically tracks the appropriateness and outcomes of patients undergoing procedures to treat blockage in the arteries of the heart. One of these procedures involves placing "stents," or small pipes, to open up areas of significant narrowing and improve blood supply to the heart. My former colleague is a fantastic doctor, and I've witnessed his impeccable medical decision-making myself on a myriad of occasions. In fact, he even trained underneath a well-respected nationally-known physician who routinely authors many of our national guideline statements on appropriateness. Appropriateness is really just a modern medical buzzword for describing whether or not a therapy is indicated for a particular patient having certain symptoms. Do you know what percentage of the heart procedures that he performed over the last year were supposedly "appropriate" according to the data submitted to the NCDR on his behalf? Do I really have to tell you? 1.8%. That's right. Supposedly, more than 98% of his procedures were not indicated and therefore deemed inappropriate. Absolutely laughable data.

This guy is the doctor whom you would want your mother to go see if she were needing treatment for her heart disease. I guess that his 1.8% still beats my 0%

regarding tobacco cessation counseling, but nearly every bit of this collected data is ridiculous. I'll even tell you why the submitted data is so terrible. I know this, because in almost every hospital that I've worked in to date, this data submission is performed by essentially the same type of person at each facility. The hospital typically assigns non-physician employees, with limited understanding of the purpose of the registry, to take on their tenth different job at the hospital, which involves filling in pages of check boxes for every procedure performed. The check boxes are found adjacent to poorly written and often inapplicable questions that the data enterer rarely even comprehends.

I want you to know that none of the individuals involved with these processes are typically bad people. Usually, they are very hard workers, trying their best. But, what I've been trying to tell you this entire chapter is that measuring quality in medicine is as complex as it gets, and despite our best efforts, no one using our current paradigm has been able to figure it out.

TIME TO THROW IN THE TOWEL

In the 1980s, Wade Boggs's fiercest challenger for Major League Baseball's batting title was arguably San Diego Padres' outfielder Tony Gwynn. Gwynn, like Boggs, would ultimately amass over 3,000 career hits and be elected to the Baseball Hall of Fame. He would win eight National League batting titles. In the six seasons mentioned previously between 1983 and 1988, Boggs had the highest batting average in Major League Baseball four times. Do you know who held this honor during the other two years? Tony Gwynn.

Although almost never actually playing against each other in the same game, Boggs and Gwynn maintained a daily rivalry throughout my childhood in the sports section of the newspaper. I'd memorize their numbers and intently follow their batting averages. Their statistics meant something to me because they could be understood. In fact, their game had the same exact rules for everyone. But, what if pitchers had thrown baseballs to Boggs and softballs to Gwynn? What if Boggs had used a bat, but Gwynn had swung a broomstick with a patch over his eye? What if either player made the All-Star Team just by buying their own awards and purchasing their own hits? What if fans, from another sport, who didn't even understand the game of baseball, were sending extraneous data from time to time to an official scorekeeper who then tried to make sense of the information? Can you imagine the futility in trying to compare batting averages in these circumstances? The players' calculated statistics would mean almost nothing.

For the last decade, I've seen us on a daily basis keep tabulating pointless quality metrics in medicine. In fact, when you research it, we've been doing it even far longer than that. For whatever reason, we keep thinking that by putting a few more variables into the healthcare quality equations, we might finally get it right. We believe that we just can't "throw the baby out with the bathwater," and that there must be some way to figure out how to make this complicated quality assessment work. The problem is that blind pursuit of this dream is leading us to destruction.

When quality measures are so flawed that they fail to represent anything close to their actual purpose, you have no choice but to throw them all out and start over. When everyone pays third parties for seals of approval, they are virtually meaningless. Poor data inputted into an equation will always equal incomprehensible data being outputted at the other end. Whenever this happens in science, you have no choice but to end the experiment. You must scrap almost everything and rebuild the paradigm. I'm so worried that you'll miss my point that I'll say it again. You have no choice but to throw nearly everything out and rethink your approach. The experiment has failed. Quality measures make no sense being interpreted like batting averages.

HOPE BY MOVING IN ANOTHER DIRECTION

In medicine, as I've told you, the variables of quality are infinite. This means that evaluating quality is as subjective as it is objective and literally there are insurmountable complexities involved. Given these circumstances, believe or not, conscious scientific assessment can actually be a waste of your time and resources. In Malcolm Gladwell's national bestselling book, *Blink*, he outlines this concept in amazing fashion. Return for a moment to think about being a student in a high school or college classroom. When you first start taking a course, how long do you think that it takes you to determine how good your professor is going to be? Do you need to hear the professor give two lectures? Do you need to sit in your professor's class for one month or the entire semester? How long will it be until you can determine the quality of your teacher?

Gladwell writes that the psychologist, Nalini Ambady, once gave her students ten-second videos of different teachers with the sound off, and found that her students had no problem coming up with an accurate rating of each teacher's effectiveness. Ambady further reduced the clips to five seconds in duration, and obtained the same results. In fact, the findings were remarkably consistent at even TWO seconds. Students viewing a silent two second video of a professor that they had never met could reach similar conclusions about a professor's quality as students who had actually taken the professor's class for the entire semester. In the *blink* of an eye, you can often make snap decisions that are every bit as good as spending a decade trying to figure them out. In fact, Gladwell argues that this phenomenon is most likely to hold true in those situations where it's impossible to truly quantify and understand every variable at play. Assessing quality in medicine is precisely one of these situations.

I'll argue that you will gain more information about the quality that I provide as a physician in 5 minutes of interacting with me during an office visit, than you will from reviewing a dictionary's worth of bogus quality metrics. Do you want to really measure quality in medicine? Schedule one person from time-to-time to come see me, unannounced, with hidden cameras, like it's a *Dateline* special investigation report, for a routine office visit. Don't give this reviewer a bunch of pre-conceived check boxes to fill out that will mean absolutely nothing. Just allow this person to write about his or her experience and post it online. Call it TripAdvisor.com. Oh, wait, that site already exists. Call it TripToTheDoctor.com. Allow my own patients to LIKE or DISLIKE the reviewer's comments, and then send a different reviewer to visit me in subsequent years to get more opinions. Finally, allow my own patients to post their reviews about me. Similar to product reviews on Amazon.com, some of these comments will be helpful and some won't. Some of my patients will blast me, while others will praise me, and in many instances there will be no true justification either way. But, some of the reviewers will help you.

I'll become just like any other business out there fighting to survive on the public's perception of quality.

Whether or not I stay in business becomes linked to the services that I'm able to provide. If I'm a really bad plumber, I won't be in business for long. People will figure me out. People will either tell their friends about my subpar services and my water well of customers will dry up in a hurry, or people will tell their friends to schedule an appointment. Every day that I show up for work, I'll be running a business, and for a business to survive, it must find a way to provide quality services. The will to stay in business is quality's greatest motivator.

The best part about this new system is that it will get rid of the old one that has been draining the life out of everyone. This new system will cost pennies in comparison to the hundreds of millions of dollars that we are currently spending on futile healthcare quality measures. What should we do with all the newfound money? How about put the resources and financial funds previously devoted to tabulating meaningless quality metrics directly back into actually enabling medical providers to do their jobs? Take all that money that we are spending to buy Accreditations and use it toward hiring more nurses to directly help with patient care in the hospital. Get rid of the third-party moochers altogether. You won't need them for quality if you return medical providers back to being the centerpiece of healthcare. In fact, even allow them to have more of a vested interest in the delivery of quality services.

Do you think that quality improvement is affected by having your name on the building? You better believe it. I have my own private practice, and my name is on the building, and that by itself drives me to deliver value because you will always be more proud of what you own or have built. However, the physician workaholic is dying. Doctors with their names on the building are fading. In fact, as I'll explain to you in detail later, with the passing of the ACA, I'm now prohibited from investing in and building my own hospital to better provide value to my Medicare patients.

The physician has been removed from the middle of the quality wheel and has been replaced by a system of check boxes because someone mistakenly felt that this would bring better quality. This will never work. Is there really any greater accountability for a physician in his relationship to his patient than the sanctity of life itself? You probably don't think about this every day, but I live it. Have you ever had to speak to a patient's family when something bad occurs to the patient? Have you ever had to explain why the outcome didn't end up being favorable? I'm not even talking about when a mistake has been made. I'm just talking about when things happen that I can't control. This conversation is polarizing and cuts into my heart too. I second guess myself. I wonder what I could have done differently. I read everything that I can find in the literature. I talk to my esteemed colleagues to learn how they would have approached a similar circumstance. Friends, the patient-physician relationship is naturally designed to stimulate ongoing quality. Just don't let your systems get in its way.

TJC has been accrediting hospital standards for more than 50 years and there is no strong data that we are any better off with our processes. You better start believing me when I tell you that this is not the answer for quality. More third-party seals of approval that you pay for yourself are not going to be the solution. Complicated systems to track meaningless quality metrics are not the answer. You don't need all this complicated mess. The bureaucracy involved with developing meaningless quality metrics is stifling. The solution to this quality dilemma, as you will see later in this book, is the physician businessman and businesswoman. In the blink of an eye you will know quality is present when this individual is allowed to return to the epicenter of healthcare. Right now, everything is backwards. You need more financially invested physicians in control of systems, not more administrators. You need some administrators, yes, and I'm friends with some fantastic hospital CEOs, but the system of quality should be built around the medical providers. The medical providers should not be placed as an afterthought on the periphery of a buggy bureaucratic square wheel. No matter how you choose to measure quality in this type of system, the wheel will never roll.

1 The Second International Study of Infarct Survival (ISIS-2) is published in the Saturday, August 13, 1988, issue of the medical journal, *The Lancet*. The article is titled "Randomised Trial of Intravenous Streptokinase, Oral Aspirin, Both, or Neither Among 17187 Cases of Suspected Acute Myocardial Infarction: ISIS-2" and is found in Volume 332, Issue 8607, on pages 349-360. An interesting side note about ISIS-2, is that the authors mention that no benefit was seen with Aspirin in the subgroups of patients born under the astrological signs of Gemini or Libra. Subgroup analysis is very common in clinical trials and involves dividing up the results of the trial by certain patient characteristics to see if benefits are consistent across those groups. Subgroup analysis is only meant to be used to generate hypotheses, because the subgroups themselves are not truly randomized groups of people, and results within subgroups can be driven by chance. The authors mention this observation regarding the trial's results and astrological signs merely to outline some of the potential limitations with drawing conclusions from subgroup analysis in clinical trials. I use this example frequently when I teach my medical students.

2 This retrospective analysis titled "Patients Treated by Cardiologists Have a Lower In-Hospital Mortality for Acute Myocardial Infarction" is published in Volume 32, Issue 4, on pages 885-889 of the *Journal of the American College of Cardiology*. Study limitations include its retrospective nature, but after statistical adjustment for patient characteristics, the in-hospital mortality reduction seen in patients being treated by a cardiologist was independent of more than 20 other relevant variables. Of note, in this analysis, the number needed to treat to see the observed benefit was 30.

CHAPTER 4:

Medical Documentation Gone Awry

"SIMPLICITY IS THE ULTIMATE
SOPHISTICATION."
—LEONARDO DA VINCI

I once worked as a resident physician at a Veteran's Administration (VA) hospital. The VA Healthcare System, at that time, was actually one of the first large medical systems to start using an electronic medical record (EMR). I've mentioned EMRs already, but an EMR is merely a computer-based system for organizing patient office visit or hospital encounter notes, lab tests, and other medical studies. An EMR is a replacement for your doctor's historic "paper chart" or those rows of filing cabinets filled with folders that had previously been so commonplace at your physician's office. Having physicians and healthcare systems implement an EMR is one of the healthcare reform measures brought forth by the Affordable Care Act, which was signed into law by President Obama in 2010. A number of people strongly believe that an EMR reduces paperwork and administrative burdens, cuts cost, reduces medical errors and most importantly, improves the quality of care. In theory, all of these things make perfect sense when viewed by the naked-eye, on a clear day, from 30,000 feet. In practice, however, the sky just always seems to be filled with a lot more clouds.

I've essentially lived out this entire EMR transition as a medical professional. When I started medical school, the hospital that I worked at was still an entirely "paper" chart-based system. As a medical student trying to learn from reading my superiors' notes in the hospital chart, I distinctly recall the difficulties that I had deciphering handwriting or even locating the results of patient labs and tests. Toward the end of my medical school training, laboratory testing and X-ray scans had made their way onto computer screens through the use of various software programs. Once I had graduated medical school and entered my residency training, EMRs were active at the two hospitals where I worked.

At that time, the VA hospital's EMR was a more robust system than the one being used by the community hospital. In fact, the VA Healthcare System's EMR was actually viewed as cutting edge technology. It not only displayed patient data in a computerized format, but this same system also enabled physicians to directly place orders for their patients, a process known as physician order-entry (POE). POE systems, which are commonplace now, were almost unheard of at that time, but believe it or not, the VA hospital had one integrated with their EMR.

The fascinating thing, however, is that this "more sophisticated system" at the VA hospital, didn't seem to make anything run more efficiently. In fact, the community hospital that I worked at ran circles around the VA hospital in terms of productivity, speed of pace, and patient volume seen per physician. One might argue that other variables contributed to the witnessed efficiency gap between the two hospitals, and indeed, I'll touch on some of these potential factors later in my book. However, I want you to know that every day that I sifted through that sophisticated EMR, I became more and more aware of the clouds capable of blocking our 30,000-foot view. In fact, almost all of those clouds are still in the way today.

The very thing that can make an EMR so robust, essentially the ease by which it's able to facilitate massive data entry and collection, is actually its Achilles' heel. The VA's EMR system only served to confirm this, and in itself, is a perfect case study for us to review. A patient would literally be in the VA hospital for three days and have 20 different notes for you to sort through in the computer chart. Most of these notes were *template generated*, which in medicine is just another term for rather *meaningless prose*. And, I'm not overstating here. All modern day EMRs are template driven, and almost every time that you request medical records from another doctor on your own patient, and you receive one of these template driven notes, the other doctor literally apologizes to you for the suboptimal content that you are receiving. There often is a standard disclaimer found within the note, as if someone's legal team has even established that the note is a pitiful attempt for medical communication. The disclaimer typically outlines something to the effect that "the note was generated by a template-based system and may or may not make any sense at all."

Regardless, there would be about 20 of these nearly meaningless notes in the patient's chart for even a short hospital stay. That's because everyone who even walked by the patient's room seemed to create a note. Documentation was the new buzz word, and the EMR system was built to be agreeable to this excessive data charting. The physical therapist, the dietician, the speech pathologist, the nurse three times a day on shift changes, the social worker, and of course the physician, were all clicking and creating one long note after another. A patient would be in the hospital for pneumonia, receiving antibiotics, with ongoing chronic management for known history of high blood pressure and diabetes. Knowing those things actually matter to patient care. But, believe it or not, this useful information was challenging to locate in the chart. Pertinent details were often buried underneath a pile of worthless database entries. You have no idea how many times that I was the on-call physician, in the middle of the night on a 30-hour shift, taking care of someone else's patient whose health had suddenly deteriorated. I remember sifting through note after note unable to figure out why a patient was even in the hospital to begin with. The clutter was overwhelming. I recall seeing time and time again that a patient was "cordial and cooperative" with "no barriers to communication" and a "pain-scale of zero" during the last nursing assessment. I could see that the patient had eaten "toast and eggs" for breakfast and "maintained no contraindications for the flu shot." But, these things were of little help to me when trying to perform serious medical assessments.

The "paper chart" had clearly hypertrophied like a muscle on steroids. Its goal was to improve function and be attractive, but interestingly, almost the opposite had happened. The pendulum had swung too far. The hypertrophied muscle was supposed to be the solution, but I ended up being more confused with what was actually going on with patients. Informative "notes" really weren't even being created at all. Fragments of thought were being pieced together by a computer system. Individual patient problems were being charted and charted again, but it had become nearly impossible to figure out how each problem intersected into a legitimate diagnosis that I was doing something about. The muscle had hypertrophied, but in the process, had somehow become stiff, inflexible, and grossly dysfunctional.

THE BLOATED ELECTRONIC MEDICAL RECORD

In the last three years, I've held the same job, in the same town, only working at two hospitals, but I've had to learn five different EMR systems. If I included my last four years in medicine, that unique EMR number would be eight. This is mainly a result of the recent dynamics in healthcare and other variables that I can't control, such as a hospital implementing one EMR, then for whatever reason, deciding to change it to something else. Most competing hospitals will not use the same EMR, and as I've already told you, I've never been a part of two EMR systems that were actually able to integrate with one another. Can you imagine learning Spanish in anticipation of a trip to Mexico, and then being sent to Italy instead? Or while in route to Rome, you learn Italian, only to have your plane make an unexpected permanent landing in Germany? This is seriously how many physicians have felt over these last several years. I've been more fortunate than most in adapting to these systems given my computer programming hobby, but I definitely empathize with my frustrated colleagues.

The point that I'm making here is that I've had exhaustive experience with numerous EMRs, and each one is infected with the same disease process that I encountered at the VA hospital over a decade ago. EMRs are *bloated*. And, for what reason? Patient care? Absolutely not. They are intentionally filled with universally unhelpful information. Every physician knows this. The system wants you to think that by being bloated you can better track quality measures in healthcare. But, you learned in the last chapter how this is an entirely meaningless endeavor, and trust me, every physician knows that as well. In truth, there really is only one reason EMRs are bloated. It's because of *medical billing*. And, if you don't listen to what I have to say in this chapter, this single parasite by itself will ultimately destroy our system. It's already placed us on life support. If we as physicians were better at organizing ourselves, we could put a stop to this nonsense. Instead, the physician workaholic is dying and the rest of us keep nodding our heads up and down at the powers that be as if we're stuck in a trance. Who keeps approving the rules for medical billing anyway? Our United States Congress? Read more about them in Chapter 8. Let me tell you, if you are a commercial insurer out there, this is where your ears should perk up. *Implement a simplified auditing strategy for physician billing, much like the one that I'll outline later in this chapter, and every physician in America will be telling patients to purchase a plan with your company.* You think that we, as physicians, can't organize? Historically, you may be right, but don't dare underestimate our influence over the hearts of our patients. Remember, when backed into a corner, patients and physicians will fight together for each other.

PHYSICIAN DOCUMENTATION GUIDELINES

I want you to imagine that you have a massive water leak in your front yard. I'm talking about a major geyser coming out the side of a red fire hydrant positioned on the corner of your lot. 500 gallons per minute of water are quickly forming a lake in your grass. The local water utility authorities arrive, and immediately begin by inspecting the grounds. They search around the back of your house, then the front, and then walk through the inside of your house. They dig a few holes in your flower beds, all the while the water continues to spew. They visit with you regarding your knowledge of any previous history of water leaks at your property. Ultimately, they examine the red fire hydrant. They document the angle of the water's trajectory and make note that its direction points toward the southeast. The authorities mention that this now qualifies as a severe leak, as tree limbs and mulch are associated with this mess. Finally, after what seems like an eternity, the authorities turn a valve and shut off the water. The hemorrhaging stops. The cracked fire hydrant cap is replaced. You wait anxiously for an update on the property damage, but the authorities must first complete a half-hour of various paperwork documenting their assessment and solution strategy. Ultimately, you are addressed by the authorities, and they answer all of your questions. You really like those guys, but you can't help but wonder what that entire charade was all about. The water was gushing from a broken pipe and they fixed it. Thank God for them, but you can't contain your curiosity. You inquire why they appeared to be doing a bunch of extraneous things. It seemed like all of that was merely wasting time that could have been better spent. The authorities smile because they absolutely agree with you. The problem, they tell you, is that no one will reimburse them for any of their effort if they don't. The system sadly only rewards things that are unnecessarily *bloated.*

You may or may not find any humor with my analogy. But, the truth remains that this is exactly what the Centers for Medicare and Medicaid Services (CMS) asks me to do on nearly three dozen patient encounters every day. CMS has actually created a 48 page document titled *Documentation Guidelines for Evaluation and*

Management Services that outlines all that I must do to receive payment. This is about the most ridiculous document in all of modern medicine. How about I just fix a leak and get paid for what I do? Nope. That would make too much sense. Instead, let's bloat the system with all kinds of nonsense. In fact, just humor me for a moment, so that I can provide you a brief glimpse into my world.

You are a new patient of mine. I haven't seen you before, but you schedule an appointment to be evaluated for fever and chest pain when you cough. Upon arrival, I ask you a few targeted questions, examine you, order an Xray, and confirm my suspicion that you have pneumonia. I give you a prescription for antibiotics. I put your medical assessment and plan in the electronic medical record. I submit to your insurance an invoice of services rendered to diagnose and treat your pneumonia, and I move on to help my next patient. That's what really should happen, but it doesn't. Here's what the *Documentation Guidelines for Evaluation and Management Services* want me to do instead.

First, I start by documenting your "Chief Complaints" of chest pain, cough, and fever. I perform what is known as a "History of Present Illness," which involves asking you a number of questions. This all makes sense up to this point. I essentially collect "points" for each type of question that I ask you. In this example, you have chest pain located on *both sides of your chest* (one point), *sharp* in discomfort (one point), *moderate in severity* (one point), lasting *seconds* (one point), and *associated with a cough* (one point). Once I've accumulated four or more points in this category, CMS will let me move on to the "Review of Systems," which arguably is the most bloated category in this game of points. A "Review of Systems" involves me quizzing you about nearly every organ that you have, regardless of whether it's even applicable to your presenting symptoms. I ask you about your *eyes* (one point) and then your *ears, nose, mouth,* and *throat* (but, for whatever reason, I only get one point total for asking about all of these). Moving down the list of systems, I then ask you questions about your *heart* (one point), your *lungs* (one point), and your *stomach* (one point). You might think that I would have acquired enough points by now to keep moving on, but I'm really just halfway there. For, this category, CMS requires me to accumulate at least 10 points! So, I continue to ask you more questions, usually entirely unrelated by this point to your situation. It's really like the water utility authorities searching the inside of your house when the fire hydrant is gushing in the front yard.

When I complete the "Review of Systems," I then obtain your "Past Medical/Surgical History," "Family History," and "Social History." All of these things are useful things in the appropriate situation, but all of them may or may not be necessary for every patient problem that is encountered. However, CMS doesn't differentiate in its guidelines for various clinical situations, so these items are necessary to be included in your note. Obtaining your "Allergies" and "List of Medications" is not even mentioned in the 48-page document, and I get no points for doing it, yet it's one of the few things that I've mentioned so far that actually should be documented.

Ultimately, I arrive to your "Physical Exam," which is second only to the "Review of Systems" as being the most bloated item in this entire process. Since you are a new patient, in order for me to receive appropriate reimbursement for the medical decision-making used in this example, I'm required to document examining at least 18 different elements in nine or more systems. Nine systems? Maybe you would benefit from having three or four of those examined for your mentioned complaint, but nine? Sometimes, depending on your illness, you may need me to examine more than twelve systems, but shouldn't that be my call and not CMS's? Ultimately, doesn't the solution matter more than the process? Do you really care how the cap is fixed on the fire hydrant, or just that the lake is gone from your front yard? The point that I'm continuing to illustrate is that CMS's required documentation strategy promotes incomprehensible inefficiency at a time when cost-effective medicine is paramount.

After completing all of the above documentation, I finally arrive to the most integral part of the entire note, my own medical decision making. This involves my assessment of your problems and my plan for addressing them. This is the only part of the note that any doctor ever reads, because it's the only part of the note that we, as physicians, know even matters. And, I'm not overstating here. I've been a medical doctor for over 10 years. I've been good friends with a myriad of other physician colleagues. I have not personally, nor have I ever witnessed any other doctor in clinical practice, read the entirety of another physician's medical note. We all just skip to the bottom and read the assessment and the plan. In fact, many physicians will even begin their note with their assessment and plan at the top, because they know that's all anyone reads anyway. The other 95% might as well be monkeys typing on a typewriter.

When I conclude my assessment and plan, the nightmare is still not over. I must then link all of your "problems" to the "Morse code" of medical billing known as the International Classification of Diseases (ICD). For CMS, we are currently using a "Clinical Modification" of the 9th reiteration of this ICD classification, which we refer to as ICD-9-CM. ICD-9-CM reportedly contains over 17,000 codes for various illnesses, patient complaints, and medical procedures. In the example above, your fever, cough, and chest pain, become known to the medical billing world as 780.6, 786.2, and 786.5, respectively. Your pneumonia code will vary based upon the type of infectious organism causing your pneumonia, but typically will range between 480 and 488, with a bunch of decimal point options for any whole number that you finally choose.

We've been in a holding pattern in the United States over the last few years regarding the implementation of the "newer generation" ICD-10 codes. I chuckle when I say "newer generation" codes, because ICD-10 has been in use throughout much of the world since the 1990s. Our situation is kind of similar to your work computer at the office still running Windows XP, with Internet Explorer 6 as your web browser. The benefit, or rather the problem, with ICD-10 is that CMS has come up with its own modification, termed ICD-10-CM, that reportedly has over 140,000 codes. I guess someone thought that the 17,000 ICD-9-CM codes that we are currently sorting through isn't enough. Regardless, if you join my world for one day, you'll know why physicians in this country have been trying to delay the implementation of ICD-10-CM codes for as long as absolutely possible. In all honestly, I'm sure the new codes will fit perfectly within our already bloated healthcare system.

To conclude my example above, the ICD-9-CM codes 780.6, 786.2, and 786.5 are finally submitted to your insurer along with a few other numbers known as Current Procedural Terminology (CPT) codes. I'm sure that I've lost your interest by now, but CPT codes exist to describe and standardize the actual medical, surgical, or diagnostic services that your physician provides you. The CPT system itself has numerous categories and reportedly around 10,000 unique codes, although I must admit, I've never counted them all myself. Honestly, I really can't keep up with all these different numbering systems on my own. Many of these codes are even prone to change from year to year, so I hire a full-time employee, who works exclusively for me, to assist in this process. At the time of writing this book, I also have two additional employees working solely for me, who assist with the documentation requirements necessary to support my medical billing. All things considered, the only way that I survive today in medicine is to have my entire operation bloated as well. I've already told you that the physician workaholic is dying, but I imagine now that it's not hard for you to see why. The cart has become too heavy to pull up the hill, and the ride down from the top just isn't what it used to be.

THE CHALLENGE TO ANYONE WILLING TO LISTEN

The next time that you hire someone in a service-driven industry to perform contract labor, I want you to do me a favor. In fact, specifically, I want you to hire a high-schooler with a part-time lawn care business to rake your leaves. But, I don't want you to pay him for raking the leaves. Instead, I only want you to pay him for *documenting the process* of raking the leaves. In fact, tell him that he must hire a few people, not to actually help with the raking, which would actually improve the efficiency of the project, but just to help keep track of everything that is going on. These extra workers can help chart things about the leaves. They can place them in categories based upon size and color. The more details that get documented about the leaves, the better chance for anyone to finally get paid. The point that I'm making is that if you can somehow convince this high-schooler to complete your insane project, do you really think that he is going to knock on your door the following year? Of course not. Your antics are going to put him out of the lawn care workforce entirely. He's going to go find something else to do. He'll probably end up going to work at Starbucks.

The worst part about one bloated healthcare note is that, more than likely, someone else is having to create a similarly bloated one on the very same patient encounter. This "double" and "triple" documentation happens all the time when you visit a hospital. In my profession, I perform many procedures in an environment similar to an operating room. A hospital nurse or technician literally documents everything that my hands do during the procedure, but for some reason, at the conclusion of the case, I'm still required to recreate my own procedure note. It's like nothing that a competent staff does even counts.

Do you know who really ends up being at the bottom of the pile in this situation? It's the family members of my patients undergoing heart catheterization (angiogram) procedures. I'm sure the family is always wondering why it's taking me so long to come and visit with them about the results of a case performed on their loved one that finished 30 minutes ago. I need to set the record straight and tell you what I'm doing. I'm usually being like a monkey on a typewriter. My procedure note literally should already be done when I scrub out of the room. There are at least four eye-witnesses (nurses or technicians) who oversee everything that I do on each procedure. If you had that many close-distance eye-witnesses for every legal dispute, there would never even be a need for a trial. My note after a heart catheterization should read "heart catheterization done and here are the findings." I shouldn't need to repeat every step of making a peanut butter and jelly sandwich for the ten-thousandth time just so I'll pass an audit on medical billing documentation.

Believe it or not, I actually worked at a hospital once where they required that I not only recreate the procedure note, but that I record the findings of the procedure THREE times for three separate systems. I literally was filling out the exact same information in three different places. When I finally decided to ask around and figure out the reason why I was having to triple document—you are going to love this—nobody at the hospital even knew. I'm dead serious. We had gotten so accustomed to bloating the system that we didn't even recognize that we were doing it anymore.

If you know anyone who works as a nurse at a hospital, I'll encourage you to go ask that person if he or she has ever witnessed or performed EXCESSIVE documentation. I'm willing to bet that this person will immediately tell you that they do it over a dozen times every day! I know this because I just asked EVERY SINGLE NURSE whom I bumped into today at two facilities the same question, and every one gave me the same answer as above. On the hospital ward, nurses literally perform their assessment by asking patients the exact same questions that I'm later required to re-ask. This kind of thing annoys me because of its inefficiency, but this ultimately annoys the patients more than anybody. Our world of relatively meaningless and repetitive documentation provides very little value to anyone, especially our patients.

Throughout this book of truth and transparency, I hope that you will recognize a familiar pattern. I'm not in the business of critiquing unsolvable problems. The healthcare system is in serious straits and we need serious people. We don't need caricatures telling us what to be afraid of or who's to blame. We don't need more people talking about the problems or remembering with longing an easier time. We need problem solvers engaged in finding serious solutions, and as you'll see time and time again in this book, the best answer isn't always the one buried within a stew of complexities.

Most big problems are solved with simple things, so I'm not going after the 140,000 different ICD-10-CM codes or the 10,000 CPT codes. I've got plenty of ideas for simplifying this process too, but I must gain momentum from winning a battle before I can contemplate winning the war. Only one thing needs to be done immediately and it deals with CMS's pointless *Documentation Guidelines for Evaluation and Management Services*. **Repeal it.** It's a doable solution that's way overdue. CMS can actually get this done in a week's time. Okay, maybe I'd give them a month, but they can replace this hopelessly outdated operating system that's staggering our physician workforce. The solution is a one page audit form for medical billing that is based entirely on a physician's medical decision making. You implement this, and the end result will be our first step toward getting all the monkeys off the typewriters.

CHAPTER 5:

Requirements for Physicians to Maintain Their Certifications

"WHEN WE ALL HELP ONE
ANOTHER, EVERYONE WINS."
—JIM STOVALL

I n my lifetime, I have taken a few standardized exams. In high school, I sat for the college admissions test, formerly known as the Scholastic

Aptitude Test (SAT), on two occasions. For medical school, I took the Medical College Admission Test (MCAT) twice. For business school, I was examined by the Graduate Management Admission Test (GMAT). During medical school, I've been administered about a dozen or more National Board of Medical Examiners "Shelf Exams." I've successfully navigated through Step 1, Step 2, and Step 3 of the United States Medical Licensing Exam (USMLE). I've taken my state's Jurisprudence Exam. I've passed the American Board of Internal Medicine (ABIM) Certification Exam, the ABIM Cardiovascular Disease Exam, and the ABIM Interventional Cardiology Exam. Most recently, I completed the Council for Certification in Cardiovascular Imaging (Nuclear Cardiology) Exam. Let's negate the numerous "mock" exams that I've taken in medical residency, fellowship, and subspecialty fellowship training, and the money spent on review courses, materials, and practice questions. Just the standardized tests listed above, in 2014 dollars, equal an investment greater than $11,000. To maintain my current four board certifications, more than $5,000 will be spent every 10 years just for the right to sit for these exams.

Testing is a part of our culture. I get that. And, I'm not the first person to question our pendulum swing toward an extreme focus on standardized testing. Ask any good public school teacher of his or her experience of being delegated by the higher authorities to "teach" a test. I even remember when I used to teach SAT preparation courses myself. Do you know the single greatest statistical predictor of SAT scores? Do you think that it's a student's grades or whether the student attends public or private school? Do you think that it's time spent on preparing for the exam or whether or not the student took a prep class? Some of those things may help, but the strongest predictor actually happens to be the income of the student's parents. That's what it used to be and I suspect that it's still the same today. The SAT might serve many purposes, but what it clearly does well is to sort kids seeking entrance into college into categories based on the wealth of their parents. Supporters of standardized testing would argue that there is a good reason for this association, but once again, that's not my purpose in writing this chapter, and therefore, I won't dwell on that debate here.

Instead, what I will tell you is that most of the public school requirements related to "teaching" a test are government-driven measures. And, as you know, there are plenty of these same government-driven regulations in healthcare. Physicians, in general, enjoy talking with each other in the dining hall about the terrifying world that has been created by the Affordable Care Act (ACA), and how absolutely no good can come from this thing. In fact, in my four years of being a physician since the act was passed into law, I'm not overstating when I tell you that I don't think that I've heard even one physician, in any dining room at any hospital that I've worked in, say *even one positive thing about the ACA*. Admittedly, that scares me a little bit. Imagine going to a water park where none of the lifeguards even want to be in the water. But, the problem isn't solely government-driven rules and regulations. Sure, a lot of ACA's goals must be modified or abandoned, and I'll specifically point out my own concerns throughout this book. However, major issues also exist within healthcare that are not a result of the government at all. These issues have been created by our own physician species.

Seriously, our medical profession has actually gotten derailed by a small group of physicians who've become so accustomed to sitting in the "Ivory Tower," that they've completely lost sight of what their commoner colleagues are trying to accomplish. Specifically, I'm talking about many of our own physician professional societies, one being the American Board of Internal Medicine, where certain physicians, typically those less busy seeing actual patients, sit around coming up with requirements for all the practicing physicians to meet. These requirements center around obtaining "Board Certifications," and then maintaining them, through processes known as maintenance of certification (MOC). These self-imposed physician regulations have become increasingly burdensome to the "real" physicians actually trying to bring quality to healthcare. Indeed, it's not just government-driven processes causing the lifeguards to get out of the water. It's a myriad of meaningless MOC requirements developed by so-called physician leadership organizations like the ABIM.

I'm not going to bore you with too many details on physician licensure and board certification processes, but I need to outline a couple of quick concepts. Think of "licensure" as the "legal" authority to be a doctor. In the United States, a medical license is issued by the state in which a physician intends to practice. In my state, the most common pathway used to obtain a medical license is as follows:

(1) Graduate from an approved medical school in the United States or Canada.

(2) Successfully pass three United States Medical Licensing Exams (USMLE), known as Step 1, Step 2, and Step 3. Step 1 and Step 2 are usually completed during medical school training. Step 3 is completed after graduating medical school.

(3) Complete one year (after graduating from medical school) of graduate medical training at an accredited program in the United States or Canada. This means one year of a "residency" or "internship."

(4) Successfully pass a medical-
legal test known as the
Jurisprudence Examination.

Once you have basically done these four things, you can apply for a "license" in my state, which becomes your legal ticket to practice medicine there. In terms of the law, you are a doctor. You can set up your own practice. You can see patients. You can perform, on your own, whatever scope of medical services that you feel that you are trained to provide as a physician. In the eyes of the law, you have reached the pinnacle. I trained an additional six years beyond my state's one-year minimum requirement of graduate medical training, but my medical license is no different than if I would have just completed a single year.

If "licensure" is a *public state park*, established by the lawmakers, "board certification" is a *private country club* with more prestigious rules of acceptance. Historically, physicians have been proud of their board certifications. You might even feel better about yourself by getting several board certifications, almost like being a member of multiple country clubs. I have four of these certifications, but don't be the least bit impressed. A few people have more. For example, within my own area of expertise, I haven't obtained board certifications in echocardiography (ultrasound of the heart), advanced heart failure, adult congenital heart disease (cardiac problems that you are born with that still might affect you as an adult), or vascular medicine, yet I treat patients using echocardiography every day, and I manage patients all the time with those specific disease processes.

For my board certification in Internal Medicine, I had to successfully complete three years of graduate medical training in Internal Medicine, or two more than my state requires for licensure. Then, I had to pass a test. For my board certification in Cardiovascular Disease, I had to first successfully complete the graduate medical training in Internal Medicine, then complete three more years of specialty training in Cardiovascular Disease, or a total of five more years than my state requires merely for medical licensure. After that, once again, I had to pass the test.

Becoming a member of a medical country club brings with it a sense of prestige. In many instances, it means that I trained longer than others to achieve this accomplishment. Most hospitals, if you decide to be employed by them, might even want you to join a country club before giving you a job or letting you do procedures at their facility. Although you don't need board certifications to be a fantastic physician, the country club opens more doors for you and provides more opportunities for medical networking.

I should make it clear that I don't dislike the idea of being in a country club. I worked hard for it, or maybe got lucky, or worked hard and got lucky, to be a member there. The problem isn't the concept of a country club or getting into the place. The problem is what I, and a myriad of other practicing physicians, are being forced to do once we make it there. You see, the country club has gotten so caught up in a members-only golf game, that it has completely lost sight of its original purpose which was to improve the quality of healthcare. Think about it. There is not one patient who actually cares what's going on inside the physician country club. The patient, ultimately, only cares what the members of the country club are doing at the *public state park*. The state park is where everyone is waiting for quality healthcare, and as you are about to learn, the country club is actually doing things to inhibit its physician members from being there.

LOSING OUR WAY INSIDE THE COUNTRY CLUB

In Luke's biblical account of the parable of the Good Samaritan, Jesus tells the story of a man who is attacked by robbers and left to die.[1] Several people pass the wounded man, scurrying by on the opposite side of the road, before finally the Good Samaritan stops to render care. Luke mentions one of the passersby who fails to help the man is a priest. Although no additional commentary is provided in Luke's account, you have to imagine that this priest is a righteous person. How could such an individual not aid an injured man? A simple explanation is that the priest is in a hurry to make it to a "more virtuous" endeavor.

Two Princeton University psychologists conducted a similar social experiment.[2] They took a group of seminary students, that is individuals studying theology in order to prepare for a career in ministry, and asked each student to prepare a short talk on a biblical theme. After preparing their lecture, the students would then walk over to a nearby building to present it. The psychologists staged the experiment such that each student, on his or her way to give the talk, would pass a person in need, slumped down, coughing and groaning. The experiment sought to determine the percentage of seminary students who would stop and help the hurting human being, and what variables were able to alter the experiment's outcome. The psychologists introduced a number of intriguing twists. For example, some of the students were actually told to lecture about the parable of the Good Samaritan. You might think that after just reading this parable and preparing an informative lecture on its divine message, seminary students would be more likely to aid a distressed person. But, believe it or not, this variable actually made no difference at all. What did seem to matter, however, is whether or not the students were in a hurry. To invoke this variable, the experimenter would look at his watch and say, "Oh, you're late. They were expecting you a few minutes ago. We'd better get moving." In fact, when told to be in a hurry, seminary students were over six times less likely to render care to the needy person. Truly, only 1 out of 10 students in a "rush" actually stopped to help. Quality human beings, devoting their lives to ministry, were literally stepping over the victim in order to hurry on their way.

The point that I'm trying to make here is that the priest and the seminary students are not necessarily bad people. They just have become so focused on their path that they have actually lost their way. The country club is supposed to be in the business of establishing a standard of quality for patients to seek out. And, in many ways, they've built a fine country club, because plenty of Good Samaritans are still members there. But, that may change, as meaningless requirements continue to mount for your physician to remain in the country club. This is important to you because, trust me, none of the burdens being placed on your physician are helping to improve your quality of healthcare. In fact, it's actually impeding physicians rendering care, and many Good Samaritans are thinking of checking out of the system entirely. A recent report[3] indicated that a majority of physicians would no longer recommend medicine as a career to their children or other young people, and this country club debacle is contributing to this dissatisfaction. Physician members are finally fed up, and unless something changes, their frustrations are going to keep impacting you.

A DIFFERENCE BETWEEN LAW AND MEDICINE

The formal pathway to becoming an attorney in the United States usually begins with attending college, for which an entry exam, such as the SAT, is typically required. In 2014, the cost of this exam is $51. Applying for law school then involves taking the Law School Admission Test (LSAT), which is $170. After law school, you proceed with the bar exam, which can be unique depending on your state, but for my own, will cost you $320. A Multi-state Professional Responsibility Examination (MPRE) might also be required, and if so, that is $80. For $621 in standardized exams, you can become an attorney. Maintaining your license involves continuing education requirements and yearly fees, but no more fees for recurring standardized exams. You've been there and done that already.

Contrast that to medicine, the other major professional degree in the United States. I outlined all the standardized exams at the start of this chapter, but I'll run the list with you again providing the cost of each test in 2014 dollars: SAT ($51), MCAT ($275), USMLE Step 1 ($580), USMLE Step 2 ($580), USMLE Step 2 Clinical Skills ($1,230), USMLE Step 3 ($800), my state's Medical Jurisprudence Exam ($61), ABIM Certification Exam ($1,365), ABIM Cardiovascular Disease Certification Exam ($2,345), and ABIM Interventional

Cardiology Certification Exam ($2,830). Not only does the combined cost of these exams exceed $10,000, the financial burden doesn't end there. Maintenance of certification involves a number of continuing medical education requirements, but also requires recurring standardized exam fees every 10 years, which for myself, includes the ABIM Recertification Exam ($1,940), ABIM Cardiovascular Disease Recertification Exam ($2,560), and ABIM Interventional Cardiology Recertification Exam ($2,560). Of those last three, I get 50% off the cheapest one, as long as I pay for all the others, but the standardized exam fee is not the only ridiculous issue.

To be honest, I'm surprised that the ABIM doesn't make you pay for a course so that you can understand all the complexities with maintaining your board certifications. Seriously, I'm not joking here. Search the web for "MOC requirements" and then click on one of the links directing you to ABIM's own website. The MOC program outline is more complicated than a biophysics class. You must collect "points," one hundred of them to be exact, every five years, but you must do at least one MOC activity every two years. You need at least 20 points in "Practice Assessment" and at least 20 points in "Medical Knowledge." Practice Assessment is obtained either through ABIM Practice Improvement Modules, of which there are twenty-two, or the Approved Quality Improvement pathway, which has fifty-two different "projects" best described as busywork. Medical Knowledge is achievable through more modules, simulators, or self-assessments. Oh, and then there is a "Patient Safety and Patient Voice" module (say what?) to complete every five years. Finally, you pay to take your standardized exams mentioned previously.

Five years ago, which is the most recent tax year available to the public, the ABIM had $42.3 million in gross receipts with $32.4 million in total assets. I actually don't even have a problem with ABIM's chair making nearly $1 million dollars per year, as long as he or she is doing a good job enabling its members to provide quality healthcare. However, sitting in an Ivory Tower justifying expensive board exam fees by claiming that it somehow costs you $4,000 through "stringent psychometric testing" to write ONE single exam test question, doesn't prove your worth to me.[4] I'm really just amazed by how little the Ivory Tower understands about how to generate quality in society. This is evident by the numerous "practice improvement projects" included in the MOC requirements. Are you serious? Every day that I go to work is a practice improvement project. I'm in private practice. I run a business. A business does not survive if it can't demonstrate value. Every day that I wake up, I start out running. I'm not certain if I'm a lion or gazelle, but it doesn't matter. If I can't outrun at least my slowest competitor, my practice will fold. My patients will go see someone else.

Honestly, the ABIM is really the one who should be performing a "practice improvement project." They may not be around for much longer if they don't. As of August 2014, more than 20,000 of its physician members have signed a petition against these ridiculous MOC requirements and are even thinking of starting their own new certification board. The Association of American Physicians & Surgeons (AAPS) has filed suit in federal court against the American Board of Medical Specialties (ABMS), essentially a parent organization of the ABIM, for restraining trade and causing a reduction in access by patients to their physicians. The suit alleges that the ABMS is imposing enormous "recertification" burdens on physicians, which are not justified by any significant improvements in patient care. Essentially, the ABIM's value is being disputed by nearly everyone within medicine, yet the ABIM thinks that I need to be performing a "practice improvement project." This organization appears to understand very little about the intrinsic value of a physician businessman or businesswoman, and actually is hampering productivity in healthcare by levying cumbersome busywork on physicians without any proven clinical value. I'll bring you more quality as a physician businessman by just showing up for work every day instead.

A BETTER SOLUTION TO THIS MAYHEM

Imagine getting a phone call from a friend asking you to make a trip to visit him. You plot out your course. You plan to take an airplane, and when it lands, you'll catch a subway, which ultimately will take you to a bus. You'll ride the bus to the rental car location, and once you've rented the car, you'll drive to the ferry. You'll take the ferry across the bay and then you'll arrive at his house. As you are getting ready to embark on your journey, a thought occurs to you. Your friend actually lives across the street. How about you just walk there instead?

The solution is not more complexity, but rather simplicity. I've already told you about easier ways to establish quality measures in healthcare, and the same philosophy holds true in this chapter as well. MOC requirements do not need to be so elaborate. Adding more variables does not equate to adding more value. Trust me, no one up in the ABIM Ivory Tower is going to be able to generate more quality for society than a physician businessman or businesswoman. In fact, in this day of healthcare transparency, how is an organization, like the ABIM, which spends $4,000 to create each physician board exam question, providing value to anyone? This is just another third party, one of many, mooching off of our healthcare system. And, if these obscene costs are being distributed to your physician provider, you can sure bet that they are indirectly being passed down to you too.

The answer to this dilemma is one of the easiest solutions to arrive at in my entire book. *Eliminate the requirements for meaningless practice improvement projects.* This busywork has never been shown to result in improved outcomes anyway. I mean, just take a quick second to really think about it. What in the world does the ABIM know about running a private practice anyway? I'll tell you: not enough. Say what you want to about our Food and Drug Administration (FDA), but if you are a pharmaceutical company, you at least have to PROVE that your drug is beneficial to someone BEFORE the FDA will let you use it. Not so with these MOC requirements. The ABIM never had to demonstrate that any of this nonsense will help patients at all. They were just allowed to think up a bunch of complex requirements, charge a lot of money to get them done, and then blindly implement self-serving strategies while pretending to protect the needs of patients. Their mistake is that they finally woke a sleeping giant.

Besides ridding the entire MOC process of futile practice improvement projects, there is also no question that the ABIM should abandon the expensive *recertification* board exams. They can keep the initial board certification exam for admission into the country club for the time being. Don't forget, standardized test-taking is a big business, and getting rid of it entirely will be very hard. For example, you already know the revenue that ABIM generates from physician testing fees. However, you might be more interested in ABIM's relationship with Pearson VUE, a professional testing subsidiary of Pearson Education, which itself is a branch of the largest commercial testing company in the world. Pearson VUE administers ABIM's standardized exams. If you really seek truth, why not inquire how much Pearson Education lobbies Washington every presidential cycle? How about millions and millions of dollars. Do you think that both the ABIM and Pearson Education have secondary gain from maintaining standardized exams? It certainly appears that way.

Regardless, let the initial ABIM board certification test, which is usually completed when a physician finishes graduate medical training, be literally the one-thousandth or so exam that your physician has taken in his or her lifetime. No further tests are likely to provide added value, and evidently they are costing too much money anyhow. Attorneys aren't retaking their bar exam every 10 years because they already know that there's no quality in a system built on expensive busywork. Medicine is no different and the time for change is now.

Physicians are already devoted to lifelong learning. It's in our very personalities. Besides, we already meet hours of continuing medical education requirements each year to maintain our legal license in medicine. We want to take the absolute best care of our patients and that goal drives each of us to remain at the top of our game. Do you know what really provides direct quality to my patients with challenging medical problems? It's me discussing their cases with several of my colleagues, allowing each colleague to weigh in based on his or her knowledge and experience. Think of this as being a problem-solving meeting of the minds, and I do this type of conference at least weekly regarding my own patients with specialists in my field. There is absolutely no better environment for fostering medical education than this one, and MOC requirements should strive to invoke a similar group-of-peers setting. I would be in favor of one open-book, open-colleague module that would need to be completed every two-years.[5] This module would count for all MOC, Continuing Medical Education, and maintenance of licensure requirements. Problem solved with simplicity. The country club is saved.

I recently received a propaganda-like flyer in the mail from the ABIM. The purpose was to sell me on ABIM's MOC measures that, as you already know, essentially no one supports. On the back of the flyer were statements regarding the results of two surveys. One statement revealed that "95% of consumers surveyed say it's important for physicians to be engaged in continuous lifelong learning and self-assessment." This one was funny to me, and I can't imagine that the results were all that shocking to anyone. This is like saying 95% of dentists feel that you should brush your teeth. What the heck are the other 5% recommending?

Obviously, we all want our doctors to continue learning as medicine evolves. In fact, as I mentioned above, this is our very nature. The second statement explained that "60% of consumers surveyed say it's very important for physicians to be tested on a regular basis." I'm sort of curious who these consumers were, because I suspect that the ABIM failed to provide them with any of the knowledge that I've outlined for you in this chapter. In fact, for the record, I conducted my own survey, which may be just as meaningless. Perhaps, I can even count it as my practice improvement project. Believe it or not, not one of my patients actually cared about me taking any more TESTS. Do you know what my patients do care about instead? They, like all of us, want simpler things. They just want me to care for them when they are sick. They want me to be available at 5 p.m. on Friday afternoon if they need me for an urgent matter. They don't want me off taking some computerized test that requires a biometric palm scan, fingerprint, and digital photograph to get in the testing center. They want me at their bedside. This is what provides more quality to them.

I want you to know that I'm not making a *request* to the ABIM to change its current MOC requirements. This is a relentless *ultimatum*, and it's not just coming from me. There are fixable solutions like the ones mentioned above, but if they aren't implemented, the ABIM is about to lose all quality-driven business-oriented physicians like myself and tens-of-thousands of other doctors who agree with me. The sleeping giant is awake. Either solve the problem or we will build our own place in the park, which is where the patients want us to be anyway.

---

[1] The parable of the Good Samaritan is found in the *New Testament* of the *Bible*, in the gospel of Luke, chapter 10, verses 25-37.

[2] As told by Malcolm Gladwell, in Chapter 4 of his best-selling book, *The Tipping Point*. The psychologists who conducted this experiment were John Darley and Daniel Batson.

[3] This 2012 survey was conducted on behalf of The Physicians Foundation by Merritt Hawkins. Over 13,575 American physicians responded, and the majority (57.9%) would not recommend medicine as a career to their children or other young people.

[4] On ABIM's website, as of August 15, 2014, under a section titled "Revenue and Expenses," ABIM informs us that it had $53.3 million in expenses in the fiscal year 2013. 38% of the expenses, or $20.3 million, was devoted to exam question development and delivery. About 18 different general/specialty board exams were administered that year, each with no more than 280 questions. Therefore, according to my calculations, the ABIM spent about $20.3 million dollars to develop and deliver a little more than 5,000 different questions, which is approximately $4,018 per question.

[5] Many physicians have already taken leadership roles in developing agreeable alternatives to the current MOC process, which includes the suggestion that I mentioned above. An organization known as Physicians for Certification Change (PCC) is at the forefront of this issue and additional information can be found about this group and their cause at http://nomoc.org. The website is produced by physician leader Dr. Paul Teirstein, the current Chief of Cardiology and Director of Interventional Cardiology for the Scripps Clinic in La Jolla, California.

CHAPTER 6:

The Stick It Where the Sun Don't Shine Act

"THE SINGLE BIGGEST PROBLEM IN
COMMUNICATION IS THE ILLUSION
THAT IT HAS TAKEN PLACE."
—GEORGE BERNARD SHAW

I n February 2013, Centers for Medicare & Medicaid Services (CMS) released the final rules and regulations for something known as the "Sunshine Act." The *Physician Payment Sunshine Act*, as it's known in its entirety, arose out of a section of the healthcare reform bill (the previously mentioned Affordable Care Act) which passed in 2010. The purpose of the Sunshine Act is to bring potential conflicts of interest to light regarding the association between certain commercial industries and medical providers like myself. Specifically, under this act, payments and gifts made to physicians and teaching hospitals by medical device and pharmaceutical companies must be made publicly available on a searchable federal database, starting in September 2014. Evidently, healthcare lawmakers think this is a good idea and believe that this will ultimately result in driving down healthcare costs.

I have absolutely no qualms with being transparent. In fact, that's precisely why I'm writing this book. To be honest, I actually find humor with the Sunshine Act, and I'll explain more about this shortly. For most physicians, however, the Sunshine Act is viewed as another lawmaker agenda created for the purpose of intimidating us. The irony is that we, as physicians, are already easily intimidated. You don't need a Sunshine Act to do that. Make a few bluffs about changing payment schemes and we sell our practices out of fear of losing them first. Ultimately, if we really became a more united physician front, silly things, like the Sunshine Act, wouldn't scare us at all. I've just started looking for ways to better unify us, but you will have to give me a little more time.

Regardless, the Sunshine Act is essentially a data dump of financial numbers linking physicians to various industries that have sought them out to be consultants or even visionaries for medical advancement. Interestingly, this isn't the only data set about your physician that's now available to the public. CMS has also joined in the game, distributing out a wealth of information dealing with physician payment and utilization for Medicare services. In fact, just in case you missed the numerous *Wall Street Journal* or *New York Times* articles in the Spring of 2014, I'll tell you that Medicare disbursed about $77 billion to over 880,000 medical providers in 2012. The fiscal year of 2012 is the only year that's been released so far, but I suspect subsequent years will follow in due time. If you get bored, you can even download multiple, exceedingly large in size, Microsoft Excel files from CMS's website. You can open the files by alphabetical listing, sort through the myriad of spreadsheets, and even tabulate the amount of money your individual doctor was paid by Medicare for that year. I'm just disappointed that CMS made the files so user unfriendly. Literally, you will probably need a supercomputer to open the files because of their size. In fact, one of the files crashed my laptop the first time that I tried to open it. The good news for you is that the *Wall Street Journal* and the *New York Times* have already done a lot of the sorting work for you, so if you trust them (I say that with a smile), you can just search for this information on their own websites.

I've really got no problem with CMS wanting to tell everyone who they are paying. I'm a little intrigued that CMS thinks that this will ultimately save money. Seems like if there were a definite cost benefit to releasing this type of information, we would have already seen GEICO and State Farm post the names and payments received by their clients who had totaled their cars in a motor vehicle accident. Regardless, like I said previously, CMS is free to do what it wants to do. Mainly, I've just never seen anyone as excited about telling you something in a language that you can't even comprehend. I mean CMS releases this now public physician financial data without so much as giving you a blueprint on how to interpret it. It's like giving me the launch protocol for some rocket mission. I don't know what to do with that information.

In fact, let's play a game for fun. Look me up on the *Wall Street Journal* website. Actually, I'll save you the trouble and I'll do it for you. Hold on for just a second. Ok, done. In 2012, Medicare paid me $122,909. The average amount paid by Medicare to a cardiologist was $223,240, but don't get caught up in the numbers yet. Let's just say that I'm less than average because in 2012, I was only beginning to build up my newly started private practice. The problem is that it's hard for you to know what to make of my $122,909 figure. Yes, the data from CMS itemizes a few things for you. It mentions types of office or hospital visits, like "Office/outpatient visit est 99214-O" and "Initial hospital care 99223-F", and it even includes the mention of a few procedures using some obscure abbreviations like "Tte w/doppler complete 93306-F". But, let's face it. This means absolutely nothing to you unless you already do what I do anyway.

While I was writing this book, Edward Snowden, former system administrator for the Central Intelligence Agency (CIA) and contractor for the National Security Agency (NSA), has been residing in Russia at an undisclosed location after being granted temporary asylum there. Snowden has been charged by the United States Department of Justice with two counts of violating the Espionage Act and theft of government property for disclosing to several media outlets thousands of classified documents that he obtained while working as a NSA contractor. In his own words, Snowden's purpose for leaking these documents was "to inform the public as to that which is done in their name and that which is done against them."

I'm not qualified to speak on the legal, ethical, or political ramifications of his actions, but a major issue with releasing to the public this type of material is that only a select few will be able to interpret it appropriately. On the surface, what you or I might think is a blatant disregard to our privacy, we possibly could view differently if we were truly knowledgeable about all the complex variables involved with our government's job of protecting us. If we had more complete understanding, we might end up feeling the same way, or we might not. But, the point is, we just don't know how to really feel until we've been able to comprehend the context of the situation surrounding the data being presented. Information without as much as a blueprint for its interpretation is meaningless.

The fact that CMS literally released its Medicare monetary data to the public without a thorough explanation of its contents is preposterous. The numbers, evidently intended for the general public, don't mean anything to the general public in their current state. I know doctors whose payments are three times mine who make my same salary. I also know physicians who have lower Medicare numbers, but whose salaries are much greater than mine. The major reasons for obvious discrepancies are: (1) this data only represents what a physician is reimbursed by Medicare (and not other commercial or cash payers), and (2) there is absolutely no mention of physician overhead related to the collection of these dollars.

Let me elaborate with a couple of examples. Since I was newer in private practice during the time represented by this data, I went on ahead and looked up several other cardiology physicians to make sure that I give you a full understanding of all the variables that CMS is so anxious to report. I'll help you make some sense out of this below.

There is a medication used commonly in cardiology to perform a stress test on someone's heart. A stress test is often needed to further evaluate symptoms that may be coming from your heart. One way to stress the heart is by exercising on a treadmill, but many patients either cannot exercise for long enough or have certain abnormalities on their resting heart tracing, known as an electrocardiogram (ECG), that makes exercising a less optimal means for assessment. Instead, these patients require a medication to simulate "stress" on their heart. One such medication is called Regadenoson (trade name is Lexiscan). A busy practice of four cardiologists may perform 750 of these Regadenoson-induced stress studies on Medicare-aged patients in one year. The cost to purchase this medication is somewhere around $215 per study, which in my example above, would result in an annual overhead cost of about $161,250 for this medication alone. Medicare reimburses about $162 for Regadenoson per study, meaning that this hypothetical practice receives $122,070 back from Medicare, covering about 75% of its total expenses for this drug. In this situation, CMS would report that the practice received over $120,000 of revenue, yet ultimately this revenue didn't even pay the bills.

In order to add more sensitivity and specificity to the evaluation of your heart, a form of imaging is frequently used. One of the most established practices is to inject a short-lasting nuclear radioisotope into your bloodstream that "lights" up areas of your heart for a camera to visualize. One of the isotopes that gives the clearest picture of your heart is known as Rubidium (Rb82). As you might imagine, Rb82 isn't available at your local grocery store. A generator for Rb82 costs between $35,000 and $40,000 and will last about one month. Then, you will need to buy another one. A well-established cardiologist with thousands of Medicare-aged patients may perform about 400 tests annually requiring the use of Rb82. Two injections of Rb82 are required per test, and Medicare reimburses about $206 per injection. If your physician is fortunate, he or she may be able to split the cost of the generator among at least three physician partners. But, even in this scenario, conservative estimates reveal that your physician's expense for each Rb82 injection is still $172. Therefore, over the course of a year, CMS may report that a single physician collected $165,000 revenue from Medicare for using Rb82, however, this is offset by nearly $138,000 of expenses. In fact, the $27,000 of net income generated is just enough to pay the electric bill along with the rent for the office space housing all this ginormous equipment. We haven't even discussed paying the salaries of the trained employees necessary to conduct these tests. Don't worry, Medicare reimburses your physician approximately $65 to spend the time reading your stress study, which perhaps can be used toward that purpose.

I could really bore you with a dozen more examples, similar to those above, found within my own field of cardiology. Mainly, I just don't want you to think that this phenomenon is unique to my area of expertise. In fact, the cost of purchasing certain medications is the major reason that specialists in ophthalmology (eye) and oncology (cancer) are generally the highest recipients of Medicare dollars. Funds credited to these physicians become more like a "pass-through," with the majority of the revenue ultimately going to pay the drug companies.

The point that I'm making here is that your well-educated and well-trained physician makes a very good living beginning later in life. There is no disputing that. In fact, I already told you this in my first chapter. My second point, though, is that CMS's release of poorly explained astronomical dollar-sign figures tied to physicians has provided essentially no benefit to the general public. The purpose of doing this hasn't been in the name of transparency, because there's been absolutely no attempt to even explain the transparent variables. This is nothing more than an undertaking to further propagate the unhealthy public perception that your physician has somehow become the greedy enemy. The irony is that I don't think that CMS is even in touch with the general public's wishes at all. I'm just not convinced that everybody out there, if you really push them to give you an answer, is all that concerned with my bottom line.

RICH DOCTOR OR POOR DOCTOR?

A friend of mine is a healthcare expert and lectures on various related topics from time to time. In many of his classes, he will often pose the following question to his students:

> "If you were to get really sick, and
> I mean very ill, would you want
> to be cared for by a *rich* doctor or
> a *poor* doctor?"

His question, to this day, still makes me chuckle. When I first heard it, I didn't even know how I would answer that one. It's like my brain was just trying to figure out what kind of social experiment I was being enrolled in. But, do you know what the most intriguing thing about this question is? It's the answer that nearly everyone ends up giving. A *rich* doctor.

I've tried to think hard about "why" people believe that. But, maybe, I don't need to think so much. It's really just engrained within our entire culture. We directly associate value with price in almost everything that we do. You want the best sound system in your car? You will pay for it. You want the best tickets to the sporting event? Ante up. And, your health is surely more valuable to you than a subwoofer and a ballgame.

In fact, be truly honest with yourself. Who do you want to be performing your brain surgery? Who are you going to entrust to remove the tumor from inside your head? You want the person trying to round a few corners and cut you a deal? You want someone with less overhead seeing patients and doing procedures out the back of a portable trailer? Probably not. Actually, don't even kid yourself. Definitely not. You associate shiny and pricey with value. You want your doctor to be as affluent as anyone that you interact with because you believe there's quality in that.

Think of it this way. You are in search of the very best person to head up a team of scientists to build a device that will solve all your problems. How are you going to find this person? Are you going to place an ad in the paper for engineers at the top of their game willing to work for $10 per hour? No way. You are going to seek out the most educated and well-respected people in the industry, and you will pay them accordingly, or risk that they'll end up developing someone else's Fortune 500 empire.

I've never met Tim Cook, current Chief Executive Officer (CEO) of Apple Inc., or Larry Page, current CEO of Google Inc., but I'd welcome the opportunity. To steal an analogy from best-selling author, Malcolm Gladwell, whom I mentioned previously in this book, they are both "outliers," defined by being "markedly different in value from the others of the sample." They are innovators that continue to help develop things that seemingly we can't live without. People literally use their smartphones while on the toilet to view a search engine that somehow keeps bringing us the very things that we ask it for. Are almost any of us the least bit concerned with Tim Cook's or Larry Page's bottom line? Do any of us dispute their net worth? Of course not. We just want them to keep designing things of quality for us.

Earlier this year, former Secretary of State, Hillary Rodham Clinton, received press for her much debated $225,000 speaking fee, allegedly paid to her to secure her appearance at a fundraiser for The University of Nevada-Las Vegas (UNLV) Foundation. Student government at UNLV even went so far as to request that she return the money to UNLV, as if the amount paid to her by private sources had anything to do with the school's recent tuition increases. This is another prime example of how skewed our perception becomes when we don't understand any of the key variables. In fact, most of us have no clue about foundations or fundraising, or how to play a hand in this world of big-booster donations. I'll include myself in the lack of knowledge group, but I'll tell you what I do know. The best tables to the event have sold out for over $20,000 each. More than $353,000 has already been collected, at the time of me writing this, through high-dollar ticket purchases. The engagement, despite Clinton's fee, or should I say really because of it, is already set to be profitable, which would be only the third time that this has occurred in the Foundation's history. The Foundation will likely achieve more of its financial goals from this year's event than any previous year. I guess that people would rather pay to hear a *rich* speaker than a *poor* one.

I want to make sure, however, that I don't get you too far off track. Money is definitely not our only motivator, even in business. We are the best at our jobs when we believe in what we are doing and when we have more flexibility and control. Money beyond a certain point actually complicates our emotional well-being. In fact, if you've already passed that point, you'll find more joy by giving the rest away. However, in almost all instances, we think of the people that have money as being successful at what they do, and believe it or not, at the end of the day, their wealth doesn't even bother us that much. "It's been my experience," Clinton said when being interviewed regarding her appearance fee, "That [people are] not worried about my speaking or my household, they're worried about their own." She's precisely right. And, that's where CMS and its meaningless data dump of financial figures has gotten it all wrong. None of us are interested in understanding this nonsense of numbers. This type of thing isn't going to do anything to cut healthcare costs. What we are seeking is far simpler than that. We want the most successful people to design our products and we want a similar group of doctors to care for us when we are sick.

THE PHYSICIAN PAYMENT SUNSHINE ACT

While I was completing my subspecialty training in interventional cardiology, I attended an educational conference sponsored by one of the major medical societies that I am still affiliated with today. It is customary for all guest speakers giving informative talks at these meetings to open with a slide outlining their "disclosures," or basically any potential conflicts of interest that could relate to the content being presented. For example, if I were going to give a lecture about the quality of food at Pizza Hut, it might be relevant for the audience to know that I held a patent on the sauce used at Papa John's. This is the type of information that you would "disclose" to the audience prior to initiating your formal presentation.

I will never forget this one lecturer whom I heard speak at the conference that year. He was an engaging gentleman. He was wicked smart, but also funny, full of stories, and someone who was not going to put me to sleep that day with only sophisticated medical talk. He began like everyone was required to do with a Disclosure slide, but he didn't have just one slide. I think that he had four of them, every one in small print, with lists of all kinds of industries to which he had various ties. He was a consultant for this and a speaker for that. He was a lead investigator for one industry-sponsored clinical study after another. He had gotten one company's grant money for this project and served on another company's medical research board. When he finished reading off his fourth Disclosure slide, he paused, and then informed the audience that if anyone else had a medical proposition for him to consider, that he would be available for a few minutes after his lecture to discuss it. Everyone laughed when they heard this comment, but I don't really think that he was joking. I just remember thinking that I liked his style.

I got an email the other day from a pharmaceutical company whose Speaker's Bureau I serve on. When you speak for a particular company in the medical industry, you are an educator to your peers. I use certain medications for indications approved for use by the United States Food and Drug Administration (FDA). I use these medications on a daily basis in my practice, and I have a wealth of knowledge about them because it's literally my job to know everything there is to know about these therapies. I'm not paid to prescribe these medications. I'm paid for my time to educate people about the benefits and the potential side effects related to their use, and to provide my clinical experience regarding their approved indications.

I've always enjoyed lecturing and educating, and despite being in private practice, I maintain Assistant Professor status at a local School of Medicine for this reason. I also serve on the Speaker's Bureau for a number of biopharmaceutical companies including

AstraZeneca, Pfizer, and Bristol-Myers Squibb, as well as the medical technology and device company, St. Jude Medical. I'm a participant in a physician advisor forum operated by Bongiovi Medical and Health Technologies, and I suspect that by the time this book is published, I may have accumulated a few other disclosures.

In the spirit of the *Physician Payment Sunshine Act* mentioned previously, I received $25,450 for numerous speaking engagements in 2013. The money that I collect is earned through my private practice and is used to cover my business expenses, including paying my employees and my own salary outlined in the first chapter of this book. You may or may not be interested in knowing that in 2013 I also received "payments" from Eli Lilly and Company, Covidien Sales, Daiichi Sankyo, Gilead Sciences, ZOLL Lifecor, Cordis, Boehringer Ingelheim Pharmaceuticals, Abbott Laboratories, and Bayer HealthCare. All of those in this last sentence, CMS lists under my name in the "Food and Beverage" category, which in my case, means that they brought lunch to both my office staff and me on a workday.

I actually appreciate the days when these companies bring food for my staff. I even try hard to make time to visit with their representatives. I suspect that if you were a farmer, this would be the equivalent of a representative from John Deere coming to visit you one day about the latest features on a particular tractor. You would probably ask some questions, maybe learn something, maybe teach the representative something to go back and tell an engineer, but I suspect that everyone would find it mutually beneficial on at least one occasion. I chuckle when critics claim that you're merely being influenced by "sales people." That's an obvious statement. Have you gotten out of bed and looked around recently? Have you ever been to the movies or turned on a television? I literally just filled up for gas on the way home. While standing at the pump, an automated message was trying to convince me to buy two bags of Doritos and a package of Oreo cookies. You can remove a salt shaker out of the ocean, but it's still going to be salt water. Might as well swim with the fish and try to learn something from it.

One thing is certain about the lunch visits. Office morale is higher on those days. In fact, I bet that if you studied it, my patients would much rather interact with my staff on the days that someone brings them lunch. You think that I'm kidding, but if you've ever worked at a place where lunch gets brought in from time to time, you'll know exactly what I mean. Most days, I'll eat the lunch. Occasionally, I'll be too busy and I won't have time. But, unlike most physicians who've become timid from the Sunshine Act, I always sign the "meal form" so that I can get charged for taking a meal. In fact, I've joked before about signing my name two or three times on the same day just for kicks. The entire exercise is just a racket to me. I presume that it's successful at keeping some honest people honest, but I've never seen that type of thing ultimately end up solving real problems.

According to CMS's data, one of the companies attributed $30.23 to my name, for a single lunch meal, in my office, on the same day. The company literally brought in deli sandwiches. Wearing shoes, I'm 5 feet 9 inches tall, and I weigh 162 pounds. I'm a cardiologist whose lifestyle is a "heart healthy" diet. There is no way that I ate more than $30 worth of sandwiches for lunch. Now, I can file a dispute with CMS, but who knows, maybe they took me up on my joke and counted me twice.

I got side-tracked from telling you about that email that I recently received from a pharmaceutical company. I happen to serve on this company's Speaker's Bureau, and the message was informing me about two recent publications related to one of its medications. One such publication was in the *Wall Street Journal*, and I had already read it, but I guess that they were sending it to me anyway. Now, here's the funny part. The email notified me that its contents, essentially the *Wall Street Journal* article, were being provided to me free of charge. Fantastic news, right? However, as required by the *Physician Payment Sunshine Act*, **a value of $9 had been assigned to this reprint** and this dollar amount was to be reported to CMS in my name. Say what? Are you kidding me? You mean to tell me that I can cut and paste an online article from the USA Today into an email message, send it to my buddy, and then claim to the world that my buddy just took $9 from my pocket? If I intend to pull off a stunt like that, I suspect my buddy would rather that I just actually mailed him the $9. But, this ridiculousness is not the pharmaceutical company's fault. They are just trying to stay compliant with more burdensome nonsense originating from the umbrella of CMS. For those of you who were fans of the American television sitcom, *Seinfeld*, you've heard of this before and it's called *The Human Fund*. In this show's ninth season, one of its characters makes up a fake charity, then hands out worthless Christmas gifts by telling his co-workers that donations have been made in their names to what is, unbeknownst to them, truly a nonexistent charity. Basically, just think up any sum of money and then claim that it's been given to me on your behalf via email. This is unbelievable. In fact, that's exactly why I should sign those "meal forms" twice. Next time, I'll tell them to send me two of the *Wall Street Journal* articles, which evidently is equivalent to me receiving $18 from them.

I want to tell you that the lecturer that day, the one who had four separate Disclosure slides, is a brilliant man. He is a consultant for all these groups of people because these groups want to pick his brain. You think that Tim Cook is just Apple's CEO? He serves on the board of directors of several organizations, including Nike. People like this advance not only their specialties, but others, because they are innovators. They provide the much needed link between the engineer and the consumer, or in healthcare, between the medicine/device and the patient's bedside. The lecturer whom I'm speaking about isn't afraid of being seen with ties to industry. In fact, he embraces it. He's not intimidated by the *Sunshine*. He is too busy being his own *Spotlight*. Metaphorically, he owns Pizza Hut, Papa John's, Dominoes, Little Caesar's, and about a dozen other restaurants. Good luck figuring out his biases. He's a physician businessman, and you'll soon learn that it's folks like him who are best equipped to solve our healthcare problems.

CHAPTER 7:

Why Your Health Insurance Sucks

"LAUGHTER IS THE BEST MEDICINE,
BUT YOUR INSURANCE ONLY COVERS
CHUCKLES, SNICKERS, AND GIGGLES."
—MARTY BUCELLA

You deal with health insurance when you go to the doctor or seek medical care at a healthcare facility. You deal with it once a year when you must select your health insurance plan from your employer. I live and interact with this world every day, and just about every day it is a miserable experience.

You really have no idea how much I talk to your insurance company. I may talk to them numerous times for even a single visit of yours. Multiply that by the two dozen or more daily patient encounters that I have and you get the picture. I hire a full-time person to spend her day doing this on my behalf and I still end up spending my own time. It's a significant indirect cost to you in your healthcare experience.

What am I talking to them about? Most of the time, it's about obtaining permission or approval to see you in order for me to receive reimbursement for your visit. I seek more approval numbers on a daily basis than members of Congress do in an election year. Imagine if you had to call American Express to get approval before using your own card to buy each item in your grocery cart. You would never buy anything that way, but that's exactly what your health insurer has me do all the time. And, if I don't play by these rules, I'll be denied payment, and every time that happens, they win.

Let me walk you through a couple real-life examples, but just remember that these are not isolated situations. They occur over and over again.

HOW THE SYSTEM WORKS

You are now middle-aged and have recently developed new symptoms of chest pain. These symptoms are concerning because they may be coming from your heart. And, since God wired all those nerves in your chest together, some connecting to your bones, muscles, stomach, throat, esophagus, lung, and yes, heart tissue, you need some additional testing to pinpoint the cause. Thankfully, it is the 21st Century, and we can evaluate whether these symptoms are life-threatening and related to your heart in a fairly non-invasive way. You need a heart stress test, which can be done in one hour's time in my office. Unfortunately for you, it is the 21st Century in America, and our health insurance system is a riddle wrapped inside of an enigma for all involved.

I order the specific heart stress test that your situation requires. Although we could do this test in my office for you today, we can't do it today, because we first need to get an approval number from your insurance company. One of my full-time office employees, who has a job entirely to do this kind of thing for you, starts the process. She gets on her computer, connects to your health insurer's website, and begins the process of inputting information about your case into the drop-down boxes on the screen. Your name, age, weight, symptoms, and portions of your medical history all get submitted, and you guessed it, the response is that your test has been denied.

This is usually when I get involved on your behalf with an appeals process known as a "Peer-to-Peer" review. Peer-to-Peer is your insurance's way of giving me a second chance, or a last opportunity, to win approval for your heart stress test by speaking with another physician who works for the insurance company. The hope for me is that this other physician, or my so-called "peer" in this process, will better understand my indication for the test, and be able to ultimately approve this study as being a necessary one for you to undergo.

I want to be clear that I have no ill-will toward any of these Peer-to-Peer physicians. In many ways, they are the last chance in rectifying an absurd process that is in place to begin with. For example, why was your heart stress test denied? Your primary care physician was worried enough about your heart that she sent you to the heart doctor in the first place. Then, I am the specialist in this area, and I felt that we needed to further evaluate you with a test, which is why I ordered it. At least two board certified physicians think that you need additional assessment for your heart, so why did your insurance company originally deny its approval?

I'll be blatantly honest. This is one reason that your insurance company sucks. They hide behind outdated policies and procedures and live by a check-box system that will never be perfect. Clinical medicine is defined by infinite variables of often utmost complexity. And, don't let anyone ever lie to you, as I've already told you medicine is still as much of an art form as it is a science. You can't simplify medicine to a bunch of check-boxes. Washington, D.C., do you hear me? You are continuing to contribute to some of this nonsense. I beg you to listen to me and give up on this ridiculousness. Train good people to make great decisions and then trust in their judgment. Put a few checks and balances in place, fine, but don't build a system reliant on the manipulation of limited and incomplete variables. This will lead to destruction, and it already has.

Getting back to my story, I obviously had no part in developing your insurance company's algorithm that was used to deny your stress test the first time. However, my experience tells me that your specific stress test was denied solely because you are 40 years old, and your insurance company does not feel that you are old enough to have heart disease to warrant the most sensitive test for its detection. Never mind that your father died at 41 years of age of a sudden heart attack after he was having these symptoms for two months. However, your insurance company didn't allow me to give them this information about your father on the first go-round. This type of data evidently didn't make their algorithm. Kind of makes you wonder what else is missing from those check-boxes, doesn't it? But wait, there is still hope for you. Remember, I get to speak to a physician "peer" on your behalf.

THE PEER-TO-PEER PROCESS

The "peers" that your insurance company usually allows me to speak with are intelligent human beings. They are always physicians, and in fact, typically still board certified in at least some type of medical specialty.

They commonly are no-longer practicing medicine full-time, and by that I mean, seeing actual patients every day. No, they work for the insurance company, which suggests that they took an exit strategy from full-time clinical medicine some time ago. They may have done it for personal reasons, or family reasons, or some of the numerous reasons that I've already outlined in this book, but one thing is for sure, no "peer" that I graduated with from medical school ever expressed ambition to go work in an office for an insurance company.

I do want to say this one more time. The physician "peer" is a smart person. I'm a smart person too. I have a degree in biochemistry, which I obtained 15 years ago. On a daily basis, however, I do nothing directly linked to basic science biochemistry. That's not what I specialize in anymore. I have a good friend that graduated with me from my college the same year with the exact same biochemistry degree. We will call him Dr. B.C.[1] He has a Ph.D. from a prestigious university and now runs his own scientific research lab. He may be the most brilliant scientific mind that I've had the opportunity to meet, and I say this not out of flattery. You go meet him yourself and you'd feel the same way about him both as a scientist and as a human being.

To your insurance company, Dr. B.C. and I are "peers," linked together by the specialty of biochemistry. But, respectfully, I know that this line of thinking is an absolute farce. Trust me, I've already told you that I'm a smart guy, but I'm no more of a peer to Dr. B.C. in biochemistry than essentially every one of your insurance company's Peer-to-Peer physicians are to me. Can you imagine Dr. B.C. being required to call me to obtain approval for a chemical that he needs to purchase in order to continue his experiments that one day may lead to the cure for a debilitating medical illness? No, this would be ridiculous. I'm fifteen years removed from the front lines of basic science research, and this is light-years away in knowledge from the specialty that Dr. B.C. is an expert.

Believe it or not, however, this type of "peer" relationship is the same one that your insurance company feels is qualified to make important decisions regarding your own health. Usually, the "peer" that I speak with is a physician with a specialty in Radiology, Emergency Medicine, Family Medicine, Internal Medicine, or Psychiatry. Most often, it has been years since the "peer" has been front and center in clinical medicine. And, remember, this "peer" hasn't seen you, examined you, talked to you, or held your hand as we discussed all possible medical options in my office. There is no relationship between you and the "peer." Yes, these individuals are smart people, but often they are no more qualified to make specialized decisions that impact your health than I'm qualified to make those same decisions for Dr. B.C.

I wish that I were making this up, but I'm not. Many of the times, the "Peer-to-Peer" physician doesn't even understand the type of technology that is now being used to diagnose or treat your illness. I once had a patient who needed a ZOLL LifeVest, which is a defibrillator worn by patients at risk for sudden cardiac arrest. That's a bunch of sophisticated talk, but just think of it as a skin-tight undershirt with a built-in electrical chip that can monitor your heart for life-threatening heart rhythms, and then shock your heart and save your life if one were to occur. My patient was young and in need of a surgical procedure to correct a severe problem that he was born with. He had already experienced two near-dying spells and was awaiting his surgery at a specialized center hundreds of miles away. He needed this protective vest immediately for a short period of time until his surgery. This device would enable him to safely remain out of the hospital until the procedure, and would actually save the insurance company thousands of dollars in hospital bills. I spoke with a "peer" that day who not only had never heard of the therapy, but had no concept of how it even worked. He wanted the patient to rent the device from a local store for a few days and then return it after wearing it for a day or two. I guess that he thought this was like a tuxedo rental. No, the patient needed a device from the medical company ZOLL, not the department store Dillard's, and the device needed to be worn not returned.

One of the more frustrating things with the "Peer-to-Peer" process is that the peer physician apparently seems to not have the power to make any legitimate decisions. It's almost as if the insurance company agrees that their "peer" physicians might routinely be out of their league and disallows them to have independent thought. Instead, the insurance company provides them with an unpublished list of a few extraneous items that, if found to be present in reviewing a patient's case, enables the "peer" physician to approve the specific request. The full content of this unpublished list is never made known, and may differ slightly from one insurance company to another. But, this list exists as I frequently hear my "peers" rummaging through it while I'm on the phone with them.

When the "peer" physicians, however, can't match anything that I'm telling them to this list, that's when the entire conversation bogs down. In fact, it's during those times that I realize more than ever that I'm dealing less with a "peer" and more with a puppet on a string who is only authorized to move in the direction that the insurance company controls. This was never more evident than during a rather bizarre conversation that I had with one of these "peer" physicians just 10 days ago. You aren't going to believe what you read, but then again, this is why your insurance company sucks.

Let's call her Dr. M.D. She is a medical director for a major insurance company, likely one of the carriers that you might have your plan with currently. In fact, if my own plan were with this specific company, I would cancel it, because I just can't imagine paying monthly premiums for this kind of nonsense thinking. Regardless, I contacted Dr. M.D., on behalf of my patient, to obtain approval for a procedure that I believed my patient needed to treat his medical condition.

My patient is about 30 years old, and I'm seeing him because he had a stroke. Thankfully, he has regained most all of his brain function, but he's at risk of this happening again. Having a stroke at that young of an age, in a patient who doesn't have high blood pressure, heart rhythm problems, high cholesterol, or diabetes, is very uncommon. Something a little odd must be going on, and indeed, it is. My patient has a hole in his heart that inappropriately creates a connection between the right and left chambers in the back of his heart. We call this hole a defect in his atrial septum. "Atrial" implies the two back chambers of the heart, and "septum" describes the tissue that normally separates these two chambers. The defect allows small blood clots to inappropriately pass into the body's arterial blood vessel system, and if the blood clot travels to the brain, this results in a stroke. My patient was born with this condition and needs to have it repaired.

Several notable people have had strokes related to this type of defect. Singer-songwriter, Bret Michaels, who first gained fame as the lead vocalist in the glam metal band *Poison*, had this occur to him. Tedy Bruschi, former New-England Patriot linebacker and three-time Super Bowl champion, and Jimmy Osmond, American singer and actor, had strokes due to this condition. This is what happened to my patient as well.

Generally speaking, there are two ways that my patient's heart defect can be closed. The first option is for me to make a tiny incision in my patient's leg and advance a small garden-hose-like catheter up to his heart. Through this catheter I can deliver a small metallic mesh device that seals the hole, and my patient could literally go home the same day with only a band-aid on his leg. The second option is for him to undergo open-heart surgery. This involves putting my patient on a breathing machine, opening his chest cavity with a surgical saw, entering the heart and stitching a patch over the hole, closing the heart, and then closing the chest wall with surgical clips. Even if there are no complications, this second approach requires a five to seven day hospital stay with weeks of additional recovery. The first option, for my patient's situation, is just as successful, far less invasive, and literally costs the insurance company one-fifth the amount of the second option. So which option does this major insurance company allow my patient to undergo? Option one? Nope. They only approve the SECOND option. Once again, you can't make this stuff up.

You would think that if there ever were to be a chance for the insurance company's medical director, Dr. M.D., to prove that she wasn't a puppet on a string, this case would be it. Admittedly, Dr. M.D.'s specialty is Emergency Medicine, and not Cardiovascular Disease, but you don't even need a medical degree for this one. Ultimately, despite our discussion, Dr. M.D. does not approve option one for my patient. It must not be one of the things on her list of papers that she keeps sifting through while I'm on the phone. I try to tell her to PUT HER PAPERS AWAY AND JUST THINK FOR A MINUTE about what she is saying. I can fix my patient's problem with literally a band-aid, but she says that only a bazooka approach is allowed by her company. A bazooka is likely not what she would want used for herself or any of her loved ones, but she's been making questionable healthcare decisions for you for long enough that she doesn't even seem bothered by how ridiculous her comments appear. The "Peer-to-Peer" process is frequently the ultimate joke and it's time we all stood up to its nonsense.

Coming back to the original case of your heart stress test, I want you to know that I won the battle for you today. Of course, the "Peer-to-Peer" physician wasn't able to use his own thinking to approve the test, but he did review the undisclosed list that he had been given of additional indications to consider, and one of these items actually matched up to a variable in your case. Your study was finally approved.

A couple of extra days have passed, but ultimately you get the test that you need. The delay involved in waiting for its approval did not kill you this time, which is good, because that has already happened to somebody somewhere. I call you with the results of your study, which indicates that indeed your heart, and not your stomach, esophagus, or lung, is the root cause of your symptoms. You will now require further evaluation, but this time slightly more invasive, with a heart catheterization at the hospital. And, you guessed it, the entire process starts again as I work to get approval for yet another needed procedure.

ROUND AND ROUND WE GO

As much of a headache as it was obtaining permission for you to have your heart stress test, I want you to know that this case was actually a less time consuming one for me. You had already seen me in my office for a visit, which typically means that my office staff had already received approval from your insurance company for me to be your doctor, even if they didn't at first trust my judgment on the test that you needed. There are many situations when just receiving approval to see you in my clinic, or believe it or not, while you are hospitalized, resemble a group of kids playing hot potato on a merry-go-round. I'll elaborate on my example from this week below, but this kind of thing will occur next week as well. It always does.

Frank is in his early 60s and comes to the emergency department for chest pain. The physician in the emergency department is concerned enough about Frank that he elects to place him in the hospital so that an Internal Medicine physician, known as a **Hospitalist**, can further evaluate Frank while in the hospital and determine the cause of his chest pain.

If working in a hospital is not what you do for a living, I just tossed around a couple of new vocabulary words that are important for you understand before we continue. Most hospitals today have Internal Medicine doctors known as Hospitalists that take care of patients while in the hospital. Previously, your local primary doctor would always have been the main physician admitting you to the hospital if you were sick. Some primary doctors have maintained their privileges in the hospital, but many of these doctors have given them up, due in part to increased time constraints from excessive administrative burdens in their own clinic. Primary doctors that have relinquished their hospital privileges must form an agreement with someone, such as a Hospitalist, to care for their own patients when they are in the hospital. Hospitalists, themselves, typically have no clinic responsibilities. They take care of acutely sick patients in the hospital, and when the patients are well enough to leave, care of the patient will return back to the primary doctor.

In the real life example above, Frank is being *admitted* to the hospital under the care of an Internal Medicine doctor known as a Hospitalist. The term, *admitted*, however, should be used loosely in this situation, as this represents the second of our vocabulary words. You would think that if you needed to be put in the hospital, this would be synonymous with you being *admitted* to the hospital. But, your insurance company prefers to make this whole hospital process more complicated. In fact, you can actually stay all night in the hospital without being *admitted* at all. You may instead be on something called *observation* status. Or, if your insurance company feels that your condition really shouldn't require you to be in the hospital at all, you may be designated an *outpatient in a bed*.

Why all the confusion? Well, your insurance company believes that some people will end up staying in the hospital for no good reason, and they don't want to pay for that two-thousand dollar a night hotel room in the hospital. And, they're partially right. Although, the majority of us don't want to spend a day more in the hospital than we absolutely need, there is a small group of people that really do seem to never want to leave. I've taken care of several of these people myself, and it is what it is. But, it's because of these few people that the rules have become so complex.

As you might imagine, there is a whole list of criteria used to determine your hospital status (*admit*, *observation*, or *outpatient in a bed*), and your status may even change during your stay. In general, the sicker that you are, the more likely that you will become full *admit* status in the eyes of your insurer. Everyone, including the hospital, gets paid more by your insurer if you are considered a full *admit*. In fact, the hospital will typically have full-time employees whose only jobs are to go through each patient's chart and see if enough criteria are fulfilled for the patient to become a full *admit*. In Frank's case, he doesn't actually meet enough criteria to be *admitted*, so instead, he is placed on *observation* status to be seen by a **Hospitalist**.

When the Hospitalist evaluates Frank, the Hospitalist determines right away that he should be seen by a heart doctor. Frank has concerning symptoms and has a prior history of known blockage in his heart arteries. I'm the only heart doctor on call for the hospital that day, so I'm contacted to see him urgently. I come evaluate Frank, make some adjustments in his medications, and run a few additional tests on his heart, which end up being favorable. Ultimately, Frank feels better after the medication adjustments, and goes home the following day with plans to follow up with me in my clinic. I submit my charges to Frank's insurance company for payment of the services that I provided him while he was in the hospital, and just this week I find out that his insurance company completely denies me payment.

Frank's insurance plan is something that is known as a Health Maintenance Organization (HMO). If you have a choice, I wouldn't recommend an HMO. You will have less flexibility when you try to find doctors. An HMO typically only allows you to be seen by a select group of physicians that have agreed to the terms of the HMO. You can't see anyone else. Moreover, an HMO will select for you a primary care physician who will act as a "gatekeeper" for all of your medical care. Without the approval of this "gatekeeper" and a subsequent referral, an HMO will usually not pay for you to see a specialist physician. The irony in Frank's case is that there is not one heart doctor in my entire town on his HMO. In fact, there is no heart doctor on Frank's HMO that even has privileges at the hospital where he went urgently for care.

Although Frank's HMO doesn't allow him to see a non-contracted physician like myself in my clinic, all HMOs, including Frank's, typically cover services provided in more emergency situations, like when you must go to the hospital. So, why didn't Frank's HMO pay me for the hospital services that I provided him that day, when I was the only heart doctor available to help him? You may have guessed it. His HMO actually claims that I needed an **approval number** to be allowed to see Frank.

The approval number his HMO is speaking about is usually one that is obtained by the hospital, indicating that Frank was in need of more urgent care. Interestingly, the hospital that Frank ended up going to urgently, which is the same hospital that called me and asked me to evaluate Frank, doesn't obtain approval numbers on patients not meeting full *admit* status. So, in Frank's case, no approval number was ever obtained. His HMO is literally using the absence of an approval number to suggest that Frank never even went to a hospital requiring urgent services, and that I forced myself upon Frank, without prior authorization, and rendered unnecessary care that should not be reimbursed. Are you kidding me?

If you are a problem solver like me, you've probably sorted through this circus and come to the conclusion that a solution might exist if I can just obtain an approval number for Frank to have been at the hospital that day. I actually tried to do this, but unfortunately, Frank's HMO doesn't allow a non-contracted physician like me to obtain an approval number. In fact, only one physician is able to do this for Frank, and it's his primary care physician, the one who has been assigned as his "gatekeeper" for all medical care.

I proceed by having my office contact Frank's primary care physician in hopes that this doctor will be able to obtain the necessary approval number from Frank's HMO. You won't believe this, or perhaps by now you actually might be expecting this, but Frank has never even seen his primary care physician. Yes, he's been assigned one. Yes, he has a "gatekeeper" of sorts, but that doctor has never even met Frank. So, what do we have here? We have a primary care physician, who has never seen Frank, who may never see Frank, and now who is working to obtain an approval number for a hospital visit that he wasn't involved in, all for what? I can't even recall anymore. Truly, it is absurdity like this that leads physicians to exit healthcare on any bus that they can find.

A SUMMARY OF THE PROBLEMS

I could literally write another thousand pages of examples like these, and maybe one day that will become another book all by itself. The problem is that your medical care is being solely driven by your insurance company and not your physician. It's as if your insurance company, for your intended trip into outer space, has selected an accountant as your skilled companion instead of a trained astronaut. Your life is in the hands of a schizophrenic system built on incomplete check-boxes that result in dangerously inconsistent practices.

The same procedure, on the same patient, for the same indication, will be approved by an insurance company one day, and denied by the same insurance company on the next day. For example, over the last year, I performed six highly-specialized heart procedures on as many patients, for the same indication, who had the same exact insurance plan. Prior to me performing the procedures, the insurance company either pre-approved them or confirmed that pre-approval was not needed. The insurance company appropriately reimbursed me for the first four cases, refused to pay me on case #5, then picked back up reimbursing me with case #6. I've appealed case #5 three different times, and each time the insurance company claims the procedure that I performed was "experimental." Really? For one, the benefits of the procedure are well-established and nowhere close to being an experiment, but two, the insurance company itself didn't feel the procedure was an experiment for the other five cases. It appears that the left hand has no clue what the right hand is even doing.

Furthermore, the fate of your health is being decided by the medical expertise of powerless "Peers" that you'll never meet and that, respectfully, are often way out of their league in a specialized healthcare environment. I have no business with my biochemistry degree overseeing the lab practices of Dr. B.C. In the same way, it should be illegal for your insurance company to operate an approval number circus, but it's not illegal, and in fact, they create that mayhem for all of us on purpose. Sure, if I were the President, I'd get rid of the "Peer-to-Peer" physicians altogether, and I'd use their salaries to pay for the studies that your real doctors know that you need. But, let's face it, that's not going to happen by tomorrow.

Ultimately, your insurance plan is going to continue to suck for all these reasons. But, a piece of the problem is actually you, and the solution begins with the realization that you've got it all backwards regarding the value that your insurance company is supposed to be providing you anyway. Remember, Frank's HMO appears to not really care about Frank at all, because if they did, they wouldn't be trying so hard to exhaust the resources of people like me who are really trying to help

Frank. There's not even a heart doctor in Frank's town on his plan! And, the only heart doctor who is available (me) is weary from circling up approval numbers from "gatekeepers" so involved in Frank's life that Frank has never even met them. Frank's ONLY hope is to learn to depend less on his insurance company, and find value in healthcare another way.

WHAT YOU CAN DO

Okay, so Frank, at some point, probably should have gone to see the primary care physician that he was assigned. Even better, he probably shouldn't have signed up for such a ridiculous plan anyway. But, don't throw your first stone yet, because I guarantee you that this charade occurs to normal people just like you every day. You don't spend the time that you should spend understanding your health insurance plan. You have the right to life, liberty, and the pursuit of happiness, yet all of those things mean nothing without your health! Your health should be your number one priority, but instead, you procrastinate reviewing the information given by your employer during open enrollment time each year. You end up defaulting to the default plan without so much as understanding anything. And, who knows, you may slide by on the coat tails of another year with great health. But, one day, if you don't watch yourself, you'll wake up and be Frank, and that's what I'm trying to help you avoid.

Your solution to this headache is to actually outsource much of this mess to someone else. For more than 99% of us out there, this is what we should do. Trust me, I've got numerous character flaws, just ask my wife. But, one that I've been working on modifying in recent years is my tendency to absolutely refuse to outsource anything. I know nothing about electricity, but 10 YouTube videos later, I'm outside climbing trees and wiring my own lighting system. I don't know a thing about water drainage, but for some reason my brain thinks that I can build a large retaining wall at my house. And, the next thing you know, I'm trying to figure out some gutter system around the perimeter. I'm not saying that I don't enjoy taking on some of my projects, but a vast majority of the time I end up doing things that would be cheaper and more time-efficient to actually delegate. I recognize that there may be upfront monetary costs with delegating, but the long-term payoff can be exponential. This is true when deciding on your health insurance plan, and even an anti-delegator like me has come to this realization. If you want to still brave these rapids yourself, maybe your technique will be better. Good luck to you. The following works for me.

My guy is Ross Gunnels. He's a life and health insurance broker who's experienced at navigating this environment. He's not the only one out there doing what he does, but he's as solid guy and as knowledgeable in this arena as I've come across. I don't care if you use him, just find someone like him.

Regardless, you need a person familiar with your local healthcare environment and the common insurance players. You need someone who will know who your network of doctors will be for any of the plans that you are considering. This person better be honest, but how the heck are you going to be able to figure that one out? Easy. There's only one test for your health insurance broker. Make sure that he or she is counseling you to make decisions about your plan based entirely on your *worst case scenario*.

If you really got sick, extremely sick, who would you want to care for you? Then, make sure that these doctors are available for you to use. You want to be able to go the Mayo Clinic, or the Cleveland Clinic, or the MD Anderson Cancer Center? Better make sure those physicians are on your list. Remember, it's your *worst case scenario*. That's the only thing that insurance is supposed to be used for anyway, and we've gotten that concept all mixed up with healthcare. You need insurance when your house burns down. You don't need it when a light bulb in the living room burns out.

The majority of people picking insurance plans base their selection on what their co-pay is going to be at the doctor's office or the pharmacy. They worry about getting this number down a few dollars for encounters that might occur a half dozen times per year at the most. Then, they end up paying thousands of more dollars on annual premiums just to have this type of plan. All for what? To save $20 on a co-pay for an office visit that was only $99 to begin with. This is absolutely ridiculous for almost every one of us.

Instead, pick a plan that will be the best for you in a *worst case scenario*. An asteroid hits you on the head and you end up spending six months in the intensive care unit on an international space station, but ultimately survive because you had the opportunity to be cared for by physicians literally out-of-this-world. Your medical bill is five million dollars. You have a high-deductible plan with inexpensive monthly premiums because you've decided that you only want to have health insurance for when disaster strikes anyway. All other times, you'd prefer to keep money in your pocket, build up your health savings account, which is essentially your tax-free nest egg to ultimately pay for the rainy day or to be used to purchase any healthcare that you find value in before you meet your deductible. Your out-of-pocket maximum for your plan is $10,000. Sure, the $10,000 is a hefty price. The good news is that you've already accumulated that in your health savings account by setting aside an extra $100 a month over the last eight years while you were training for that space flight. Even if you didn't have the funds available, $10,000 is a used car purchase, and you've managed to pay off two of those vehicles in the last decade anyway. You can make those payments. And, the best thing, besides still being alive, is that your *worst case scenario* plan pays the other $4.99 million!

I'll tell you another true story. There once was a guy whose wife was pregnant. Two options existed for him regarding his wife's planned hospital delivery of their son. He could change the family insurance plan to one with much higher monthly premiums that included maternity benefits, or keep his same plan, save on the monthly premiums, and pay out-of-pocket for all incurred delivery expenses until his out-of-pocket policy maximum was reached. This guy was very smart, so he called local competing hospitals and obtained their reduced cash price for hospital labor and delivery. After adding up a few numbers, he decided to keep his current plan and pay cash for labor and delivery at the hospital that he felt provided him the best value. No maternity plan was added. And, do you know what ultimately happened? He saved his family $7,000.

Look, this type of plan may not be the best option for you, but that's why you've got Ross to help you out. He'll let you know what best fits your situation. But, for most people, this will end up being a plan that you'll only use in your *worst case scenario*. The rest of the time, you'll be saving money that ultimately can be used toward purchasing more valued healthcare services. What do I mean by this? I mean that you should use what's saved up in your health savings account to buy what you need on a daily basis with healthcare. This way, you can seek out the best value for your weekly allergy shots in town. You can choose the best pharmacy to get your medication filled. You'll only use your insurance when a meteor shower causes you to meet your deductible, and your *worst case scenario* will actually be something that you've already prepared for and built everything around anyhow. Furthermore, your approach will encourage the business-oriented physician to thrive, which you'll later learn is a solution to our healthcare crisis.

You ever wonder why doctors don't routinely display their pricing for individual services? Think about it. Every product advertisement that you see usually lists a price of some kind on it. Why don't all physicians advertise theirs? Do they think that their price would be viewed as too high or too low? Mercedes-Benz almost proudly demonstrates online that their 2014 S-Class Sedan starts at just over $94,000. Click on the image and one page after another shows you all the value that you get for that price. Walmart advertises on their website that they've rolled back the cost of photo stationary to 70 cents. Those are examples of both sides of the spectrum letting you know how valuable their products are to you.

If you are a physician out there, I challenge you to become a physician businessman or businesswoman and make your cash price of services easily available to potential patients. It's like posting your hospital's emergency department wait times on a billboard, or the number of days it takes for a new patient to get in to see a primary care physician in your large healthcare system. Why not? What are you afraid will happen? You'll learn even more about the helpful roles of physician businessmen and businesswomen in the later chapters of this book, but why not let your front desk staff disseminate pricing information over the phone, or better yet, post your fees for services on your website. Naysayers will try and tell you that the general public isn't smart enough to understand value in healthcare. They will tell you that somehow patients will migrate unsuspectedly to bad physicians offering lower cost, but suboptimal, services which ultimately will result in harm to the public. It's another poor example of someone trying to save you from yourself. Don't buy into this nonsense. Do you really think that someone is going to get their heart operated on by just anyone with a price tag on their door? Of course not. People will do what they always do. They'll rely on past experiences, they'll ask a buddy or a family member, or turn to a well-respected maven in town to help them determine where valued services are found. Capitalism itself creates its own spectrum of value as long as the user of the product is ultimately the one buying it. Don't worry, people will be able to determine value in healthcare, because this is what they do. We are constantly making value assessments every day of our lives. Mercedes-Benz wants you to believe that they are "the best or nothing," and maybe they are that to you, but ultimately it's my own decision to make, and I've chosen to drive a Ford.

---

[1] I've changed this person's name and identifying details.

CHAPTER 8:

The Physician Businessman

"YOU'RE GENERALLY BETTER OFF
STICKING WITH WHAT YOU KNOW."
—DONALD TRUMP

Mehmet Cengiz Oz was born in the American midwest, the son of Turkish immigrants to the United States. He graduated from Harvard University in the early 1980s and received his Doctor of Medicine (M.D.) and Masters in Business Administration (M.B.A.) degrees from University of Pennsylvania School of Medicine and The Wharton School of Business. He would complete lengthy training in the medical subspecialty of cardiothoracic surgery and has been a professor of surgery at Columbia University in New York since 2001. But, you really don't know him for any of those accomplishments. You know him as Dr. "Oz."

Dr. Oz first appeared on *The Oprah Winfrey Show* in 2004 and shortly thereafter gained international recognition as the show's health expert. In 2009, he began hosting his own show, *The Dr. Oz Show*, a television program focusing on medical issues and personal health, which is now in its fifth season. Dr. Oz has founded or co-founded a number of corporations, received several patents, authored numerous research papers and books, and also hosts a talk show on Sirius XM Radio. Dr. Oz is a physician businessman.

I've never met Dr. Oz. Before writing this, I had never seen one of his shows or read any of his books. I have no idea if he's really a good guy or not. But, here's what I do know. He has always been well-liked. He was Class President in college, and President of the Student Body in medical school, and you aren't elected to these positions without being popular. Everyone that I knew who watched *The Oprah Winfrey Show* loved him, and we all know that show had a ton of fans. If you believe in education, he's a brilliant man, with degrees from our nation's most well-respected institutions. Yes, like arguably every successful individual including Bill Gates (read Malcolm Gladwell's bestselling book *Outliers*), Dr. Oz has had his share of "luck" along the way, but Dr. Oz has also earned his platform of being medical visionary and consultant.

The truth is that you don't get to where Dr. Oz is today without becoming controversial at some level. For example, he is a proponent of alternative and complementary medicine, a term used to describe therapies that are often considered less mainstream in the United States, and some of his show's content has been criticized as being "non-scientific." He recently appeared before a Congressional hearing on consumer protection related to this type of criticism. Part of this criticism was directed toward Dr. Oz's prior endorsement on his show of Green Coffee Beans as a weight-loss miracle supplement.

The Senate committee felt that presumably unsubstantiated claims like this by Dr. Oz, whether it be intentional or not, perpetuate potential scams on the American public. Put more simply, if Dr. Oz tells you that Green Coffee Beans are helpful, and an unregulated third-party, with no ties to Dr. Oz, begins to market a product as containing Green Coffee Beans using Dr. Oz's own words, the American public may be harmed. Of course, the Senators failed to address the major issue of the unregulated vitamin and supplement industry, which allows for a company to market a product *as containing Green Coffee Beans* without that company actually having to demonstrate to the public that *it contains Green Coffee Beans*.

But, this still doesn't answer the question, are Green Coffee Beans even helpful? Dr. Oz evidently thinks so. Yet, why are his comments being criticized as "non-scientific?" This next discussion is also another book in itself, but I'll summarize what you need to understand in order to see where I'm going with this.

THE UNCERTAINTY OF SCIENCE

We, the scientific community, have arbitrarily drawn a number in the sand to help us to decide what is proven fact and what is not. That number is 95%. That means that for any of our medical studies to show benefit, we must statistically prove it with greater than 95% certainty. We might not say it exactly like that, because we prefer technical terms like p-values and other statistical mumbo-jumbo to make it all sound complex, but trust me, this is what we really mean. If we statistically achieve greater than 95% certainty in a study, the headline for the *Wall Street Journal* will usually be positive and state: "Medicine Works!" If we don't, then the headline will be negative and proclaim: "Medicine Fails!"

Now, what if the medicine we are testing shows a strong trend toward benefit but with only 90% certainty? Well, like I told you already, that headline will be "Medicine Fails!" because we weren't more than 95% sure. But, aren't we still 90% certain that this medicine will help you? Well, yes, statistically, we are, but for whatever reason that's just not good enough for us to prove it as fact. However, if you were really ill, and nothing mainstream had helped you, and I was a brilliant guy and 90% sure that a particular medicine would benefit you, would you have hope again and consider giving it a try? Well, the Senate committee would prefer that you not do this type of thing on the basis of it being "non-scientific."

For the record, medical studies aren't just limited by the 95% rule. There are all types of limitations to even our best science if you really want to dig deep to find it. One more example is that the data collected from the majority of medical studies that you read about is analyzed using an intention-to-treat analysis. This is another vocabulary word, but I'll quickly bring this concept to life for you.

You enroll people in a study by placing them in two groups, Group A and Group B. You assign individuals in Group A to take Medicine A, because you really do *intend* for them to be treated with Medicine A. You assign individuals in Group B to take Medicine B, because you really do *intend* for them to be treated with Medicine B. This should work perfectly, right? However, as you might expect, in real life all variables can never be completely predicted or controlled. What inevitably happens in nearly every study is that for whatever reason some of the people in Group A don't actually end up taking Medicine A. I realize that this seems a bit odd to you if you aren't accustomed to medical studies, but this happens all the time. Occasionally, a patient in Group A will just decide not to take Medicine A. Or, maybe a patient in Group A, who hasn't even started his/her first dose of Medicine A, has an adverse event. In both of these circumstances, Medicine A is clearly not the cause of the adverse event, but in an intention-to-treat analysis, this counts against Medicine A. Even more bizarre is when a patient in Group A on Medicine A is switched for whatever reason by his/her physician midway through the study to Medicine B. Now, when this patient has an adverse event on Medicine B, you guessed it, with an intention-to-treat analysis, this adverse event gets recorded against Medicine A, solely because the patient was originally *intended* to be treated with Medicine A. Unbelievable, but true. How can this craziness happen, you ask? Well, it does, and it's more common in clinical trials than you think.

The point that I'm making here is that medical studies are challenging to organize and conduct. Variables are immense and difficult to entirely control, and unpredictability abounds. Ultimately, you have to come up with some agreed-upon way to analyze the data, but since there is no perfect way, limitations will always exist, and in many cases, results aren't even reproducible. You see, what the Senators believe to be "scientific," Dr. Oz knows is just a best guess anyhow. Dr. Oz is about three mental steps ahead of the Senators, which actually makes the entire Congressional hearing somewhat humorous. It's like having someone who once read a book about a piano, question Mozart about the selection of notes in his Symphony #40.

One particular Senator was dramatically concerned about the "false hope" that Dr. Oz's rhetoric provided viewers. Another comment questioned why Dr. Oz did not use his show to promote what actually has been proven to help people lose weight—careful eating and exercise. "I want to see all that floweriness, all that passion, about the beauty of a walk at sunset," the Senator said to Dr. Oz.

Respectfully, Senator, I'm at least 90% certain that Dr. Oz has provided more hope to more people than the Federal Trade Commission. And, regarding a walk in the sunset, you should read what Dr. Oz has to say about that one in his best-selling book *YOU: On a Walk*. The Senate committee has it all backwards. Dr. Oz is the solution, not the problem.

THE SCIENCE BEHIND GREEN COFFEE BEANS

I keep dodging the question about the Green Coffee Beans. Are they helpful? As in turns out, somewhat contrary to some of the Senators' comments, there is some "scientific" data about those beans. In fact, with greater than 95% certainty, a study in 2012 demonstrated an average 18 pound weight loss over 22 weeks by taking a Green Coffee extract product.[1] One critique of this study would be that it only enrolled 16 patients, so perhaps a larger scale trial should be performed.

If you'd like to temper the enthusiasm for Green Coffee Beans, you might site a 2013 publication suggesting that chlorogenic acid, the main ingredient in these coffee beans, did not appear to be beneficial and was associated with increasing insulin resistance, which can be thought of as being a precursor for developing diabetes.[2] The critique on this study would be that it was done in (don't laugh) mice, so we have absolutely no idea what the heck it would really have done for the human species.

Finally, if you wanted to pool together a group of studies, referred to as a meta-analysis, in order to look at larger patient numbers than what a single study might be able to evaluate, you would be interested in an article published in 2011. This meta-analysis of three clinical trials evaluating a total of 142 patients concluded that an average weight loss of 5.4 pounds was seen in individuals treated with Green Coffee extract verses placebo (or "sham" therapy). And, for the record, the modest weight loss benefit seen in these individuals was deemed to have occurred with greater than 95% statistical certainty.[3]

PHYSICIAN BUSINESSMEN AND BUSINESSWOMEN AS A SOLUTION

Maybe Dr. Oz has the answer, maybe he doesn't. But, it's physician businessmen and businesswomen like him that are most equipped to save our healthcare system. In business, you have no product if there is no value. In healthcare, the problem is that few perceive it as valuable anymore. The solution is people like Dr. Oz. He has somehow found a way to re-associate worth with medicine. The *Dr. Oz Show* exudes a usefulness to the general public whether you like it or not. It has been nominated for several awards, and Dr. Oz has won multiple Emmys. People tune in because they get something out of it. There is only one thing that I know with certainty, and I'll make this point crystal clear in the upcoming chapter: physician businessmen and businesswomen are the people capable of putting value back into healthcare.

1 The study, titled "Randomized, double-blind, placebo-controlled, linear dose, crossover study to evaluate the efficacy and safety of a green coffee bean extract in overweight subjects," is published in the medical journal, *Diabetes, Metabolic Syndrome and Obesity: Targets and Therapy*, 2012, Volume 5, pages 21-27.

2 This publication, titled "Supplementation of a high-fat diet with chlorogenic acid is associated with insulin resistance and hepatic lipid accumulation in mice," is published on pages 4371-4378 in the May 8, 2013 issue of the *Journal of Agriculture and Food Chemistry*.

3 This meta-analysis, titled "The Use of Green Coffee Extract as a Weight Loss Supplement: A Systematic Review and Meta-Analysis of Randomised Clinical Trials," is published in the 2011 Volume of *Gastroenterology Research and Practice* (Article ID 382852, 6 pages).

CHAPTER 9:

Restoring Value to Healthcare

"IT IS NOT THE STRONGEST OF THE SPECIES
THAT SURVIVES, NOR THE MOST
INTELLIGENT, BUT THE ONE MOST
RESPONSIVE TO CHANGE."
—CHARLES DARWIN

T here are three hospital systems within 15 miles of my house. In the last year, one of these systems merged with a larger one to form a mega-healthcare system. The second hospital system was recently purchased by another national giant that has over $10 billion in annual revenue. The third hospital is already owned by a Fortune 500 company that operates over 200 hospitals. Indeed, the current trend has been for healthcare systems to garner more critical mass by becoming larger and larger, but unfortunately, this isn't the solution to our crisis. As you already know by now, the crisis is one of value, and perhaps contrary to what you might think, larger doesn't always equate to value added, and this is especially true in healthcare.

I've had the opportunity to work at seven different hospital systems in four different towns over the last decade. I once tried to add value to one of these systems by revamping a portion of its website to aid in recruiting. I built what others thought was a fantastic subdomain webpage. To use my own website as an example, if ecgsource.com is the domain name, a subdomain might be recruiting.ecgsource.com. Basically, it's just a secondary page or department found within the company's main website. My new website had a modern layout with 21st century color schemes and multimedia. Everybody that I spoke to agreed it was 100 times better in look and content than the current site. But the healthcare system that I built it for never ended up even using it. They kept using the old one, because ultimately the corporate office decided that all of their webpages must maintain the exact same look and feel. This meant that every subdomain had to be comparable in layout to the main homepage. Makes perfect sense, right? Why add value with newfound content and creativity when you can keep everything looking mundane? I never understood this one.

I chaired a committee at a hospital once where a respected physician complained at one of our meetings that he was having difficulty finding pre-printed order sets on the hospital ward. This was back in the day when physicians still submitted written orders on a piece of paper (instead of computer-based entry as it usually is now) to get tasks done for patients. There were essentially pieces of paper with various orders on them for various patient conditions. For example, if you were admitted to the hospital with pneumonia, there might be a physician order set for pneumonia that would have various orders on it that applied to your illness. Multiple printed copies of these order sets were found in pull-out drawers throughout the hospital, or inconsistently as files in folders on certain computers. However, the organizational system was a nightmare, and there was no centralized location to search and locate what you needed quickly.

In response to this physician's concerns, I suggested to the administrators on the committee that we put these order set files on an internal hospital website so that you could download them from any computer on the hospital ward. I told them that if I could just obtain momentary access to the hospital's web server, I'd develop a webpage with all of the content and then incorporate an easy to use search bar for finding all the files. I told them that I'd have everything fixed in the morning. They told me that this couldn't happen because the corporate office would be against these local modifications of the website. Are you serious? They would really be against adding value? You can't make this stuff up.

Once, I worked within a healthcare system that had a fantastic electronic medical record (EMR). Now, that's an oxymoron, because absolutely no one ever thinks an EMR is fantastic, but this one really was. The reason why is because it was actually developed and hardcoded by a physician businessman. In fact, this guy used to write code for games from the original Commodore 64 computer. Then, he became a physician and used his computer programming knowledge to develop an EMR all by himself. And, he was so far ahead of the curve that he did all of this long before the term, EMR, was even commonplace. The EMR was absolutely fantastic and he was constantly adding updates and improvements to match the dynamic environment of medicine.

So what happened to this incredible EMR? Well, you won't believe this, but ultimately, the large healthcare system that it was built for let this guy actually go and then they bought a different EMR that was absolutely terrible. It was so terrible that they have since bought another one. So, why did they let this guy and his EMR system get away? Oh, I'm sure that they'd give you lots of reasons that still wouldn't make any sense, but I'll tell you the real one: despite what they'd like you to believe, most large corporations frown upon a single powerful and innovative employee. It's almost as if they'd prefer their employees to have no identity, remain mediocre, and not outshine the corporation. Value often gets crushed within corporations, not added.

(I'll take an aside for a moment, because I want to make it clear that I'm not against all big businesses. Case in point: I've never worked for Apple or Google, so I really don't know anything about the internal workings of these two corporations. But, I think that there is a chance that they've found a way to allow for their workers to maintain their innovative nature and creativity. The only reason that I suspect this is because most of us actually find value in their products. My experience with healthcare systems, in general, however, is that they are way behind the curve in this matter.)

Sometimes, the greatest obstacle for larger healthcare systems in creating value is that frequently their corporate office and acting decision maker is no less than five states removed from the local environment. I once knew a higher-level administrator at one of these "spoke" hospitals within a large healthcare system. She required approval from the main corporate location before a local purchase order of over $6,000 could be made. Really? Hospitals have millions of dollars per month budgets. That's like my wife needing to confer with me before buying anything at the grocery store that costs more than a can of peaches. Why even have a local CEO if every little decision is still being made from the main headquarters? Shortly thereafter, the CEO of this hospital left, which was one thing that actually made sense to me.

I did medical procedures at a hospital once that had problems with cellular phone and data reception inside their cardiac catheterization lab. This was a major problem, because when I was scrubbed in doing a procedure in this lab, you had difficulty getting a hold of me in emergent situations. I told the hospital about the situation and I also told them about an easy solution, which involved purchasing a small signal booster for the lab. In fact, I had just purchased one of these signal boosters for my home for similar reasons, and it worked fantastically to solve the problem.

For more than 10 months, the hospital hemmed and hawed about this situation. I have no idea what they were really doing, but they truly gave every indication that they were continuously working on this issue for me. Initially, there was a problem with a purchase order. Then, because they had recently changed vendors for this kind of thing, they were working toward finalizing a new contract with a new company. Finally, they told me that it was fixed, and I went back to do a procedure there and missed six messages during a 45 minute case. To this day, the problem has not been fixed, but they claim to still be working on it. All of this, I repeat, could be solved by me with a couple hundred dollar signal booster if they would just allow me to install it.

On more than one occasion in the past, I have attempted to provide value to a hospital by discussing with its administrators feedback that I had received from my own patients related to their facility. There were simple areas for improvement dealing with room cleanliness and minor modifications that could be made with patient scheduling and hospital flow to allow patients to have more of a personalized and "club-like" experience for their healthcare. I even provided examples of how minimal structural renovations would assist their facility in a competitive local environment, and how best to go about with these improvements. How did that play out? Well, my patients tell me the same problems that were present back then are evidently still there today, and the hospital's market share continues to decline.

Concerns with inappropriate and unnecessary medical testing have contributed to a loss of trust in our healthcare system. And, as you might imagine, without trust, value suffers greatly. I once designed a web-based module that could easily guide physicians into ordering the most appropriate heart stress tests for their patients. This module was simple, yet robust, and would provide enhanced value for the system by preventing unnecessary and costly studies. My module was presented to one of the large healthcare systems that I was working within at the time, and all agreed on its value, yet I'm still waiting to hear back about the possibilities of its implementation. Again, the point that should be apparent to you by now is that a healthcare bureaucracy thinks value exists in procedures and policies, but in most instances this merely delays or crushes innovation and creativity.

I presented my ECGsource.com idea to a major healthcare system prior to its development. In this case, the powers that be were actually fired up about an idea that could assist in growing their vision of being a provider of medical education. I understood the plan to be for the information technology, media, and marketing departments of this large corporation to work alongside me in bringing this concept to fruition. I waited and waited. More meetings and more coffee that I don't drink, but no real progress. Perhaps, had I given it a decade more with this company, we might have finally put something together. But, ultimately I gave up waiting on a large healthcare system to steer its tanker ship. I chose myself instead, developed everything, completed the project in six months, and launched with essentially no one else's help. Are you getting this?

Literally, I could go on and on with stories of futility dealing with my attempt to improve the perceived value of large healthcare systems. In fact, these are just the ones that popped into my head during the last 30 minutes when I was on a jog. But, don't let all these stories cause you to lose sight of my simple point. The point really is that if you're a patient out there, or might ever be one in the future, I'm so passionate about this because of you. You see, a tanker ship is where your healthcare system is headed to unless you call up your Senator and tell her that she's got it all backwards. Dr. Oz is not the problem. Put no focus there. Tell her that a small tugboat can outmaneuver a large tanker ship every time. The solution is not more tanker ships, it's more tugboats, captained by physician businessmen and businesswomen. And, the best way that your Senator can help you is to quit creating waves that interfere with these tugboats.

THE VETERAN'S ADMINISTRATION

You still not convinced? Think about perhaps the biggest tanker ship in our healthcare system. In fact it's so big, it's like an aircraft carrier. It's the Veteran's Administration (VA). God bless our Veterans. I take care of many of them when their closest hospital to me (about an hour and a half away) is full. That's one case when the government authorizes the veterans in my community to receive care at a non-VA and much more convenient local hospital. Good luck getting reimbursed by the VA in a timely fashion being an out-of-network private practice physician, but who cares, I'd take care of these folks for free anyway. And, many times I do.

Previously, as you already know, I worked at a VA hospital facility. In case that you fell asleep for the entire first half of 2014, you may have missed some of the saga of the VA Healthcare system, which has come under fire recently for allegations of corruption, systemic fraud, and dangerous inefficiencies. I'm not here to discuss any of the criminal allegations against some of its high-level physicians and employees. I never witnessed anything illegal in my short interaction with that system. Moreover, I want to emphasize that I know some very good people, physicians included, still working in that system, and I feel for them right now, because in no way do these allegations undermine the excellent care that they have provided and will continue to provide to our veterans.

But, I'm here to be transparent, so I'll continue to be honest. I didn't want to work in that system back then and I don't want to work there now. Too much bureaucracy. Actually, it's a like a bureaucracy on steroids, and if you've learned one thing from me in this book, it's that policies and procedures don't necessarily equate to value. And, if some of these criminal accusations prove to be truthful, that just proves to me that all this paperwork doesn't do a dang thing to prevent corruption either. My worst fear is that whoever is appointed to revamp this system does what often happens in these situations: he or she comes in and establishes more policies and procedures. In fact, do you know what I would do if I ever became CEO of a large healthcare system? Every day that I showed up for work, I would make it a point to get rid of at least one pointless policy. Why? Because policies bog down tugboats that are trying to be innovative and add value.

Yes, you have to maintain some structure to every system, but policies created at meetings by individuals who have no contact with the front line of patient care should be expunged, because there is not value in this type of thing.

You could have asked me or any of my physician colleagues that worked at that VA hospital if there were inefficiencies that needed to be addressed, and we all would have agreed on the system's myriad of problems even back then. In fact, you could probably ask any physician that has worked even briefly in the VA Healthcare System over the last 30 years the same question, and you would get an identical answer. How do I know this? Because I've asked these folks myself, and they've told me the same thing. Healthcare is a dynamic environment. The best medical therapy or test today is probably not going to be the best one tomorrow. Treatments are so rapidly evolving that even guideline statements put out by major medical societies are having trouble keeping up with all the new publications. Don't you see what the major problem is here? It's the one that our VA Healthcare System so clearly uncovered. The fog has been lifted, but tanker ships are not designed to steer.

WHY NOT BUILD MY OWN HOSPITAL?

From all the things that I've told about large healthcare systems and the obstacles these institutions must overcome to provide you value, you'd probably think that I should just buy my own hospital. If I did that, you are correct in thinking that I could eliminate many of the problems that I outlined to you above. My hospital could be managed much as I do my own private practice clinic. Meaning, that if my website needed to provide you more value, I'd just update it without a bunch of red-tape involved. If you came to see me for a visit and mentioned that my floor was dirty, I would call the cleaning company that night. If our cell phone reception was suboptimal and you were missing important business calls while at my facility, I'd walk down the street to the store and pick up a $200 signal booster and it would be installed by the afternoon. I could do these things for you in my own hospital almost the same as I already do for you in my clinic. Remember, I'm a physician businessman, and I understand value.

One obvious problem with this plan is that I don't have tens of millions of dollars right now to buy and staff this hospital. The second issue is that my own members of Congress are working extremely hard to make this illegal for me to do. Generally speaking, federal and state laws enacted over the last several decades have sought to restrict or regulate physician ownership of these type of facilities. These restrictions exist predominantly due to three major legislative efforts: (1) "Stark Laws," (2) certificate of need laws, and (3) most recently, the Patient Protection and Affordable Care Act (ACA).

The "Stark Law," as it has become known, was introduced by former United States Representative, Pete Stark, and was passed by Congress originally in 1989. The initial point of this law was to regulate physician referrals of Medicare patients to physician-owned labs and services, something known as self-referrals. As I've told you, government-funded Medicare is the largest health insurer in the United States, typically processing over one billion annual claims. This Stark Law was created after research showed that physicians who owned physical therapy or laboratory facilities referred patients for these services at much higher rates than other physicians. Basically, if I own my own barber shop, I'm more likely to recommend that you get your hair cut by me on a scheduled basis. The government was upset by this concept, and with subsequent amendments over time, this law has been expanded to include additional medical services such as home health, radiology services, and inpatient and outpatient hospital services.

But, I know what you are thinking. You believe that you've heard of, or read about, or even been to some hospital that you thought was physician-owned. How can this be? Are such hospitals operating illegally? Well, as it turns out, there are a number of exemptions that pertain to the Stark Laws. For example, these laws do not ban physician self-referrals to ambulatory surgical centers (more on these outpatient medical facilities will come shortly), specialty hospitals, or to services provided within a physician's practice. Initially, there was even a "Whole Hospital Exemption" allowing physicians to have ownership in an entire hospital facility as long as it wasn't just part of the facility or services provided.

Due to some of these exemptions outlined above, in 2013, according to the Physician Hospitals of America, more than 235 hospitals were owned by doctors scattered around 33 states in the United States. They are especially prevalent in Texas, Louisiana, Oklahoma, California, and Kansas. Why these states? Well, the answer lies in understanding the second of the three legislative efforts mentioned above, certificate of need laws.

The purpose of certificate of need (CON) laws are to eliminate duplication of certain resources, such as preventing 10 electric companies from trying to operate the same neighborhood. CON laws related to healthcare govern new construction and expansion of hospitals and the purchase of expensive equipment. If you can't demonstrate a need for these healthcare services in your area, then you can't get a permit to build your hospital there. These laws, in general, tend to be more state-specific, and states with weak or no CON laws (such as Texas) typically will have more types of specialty hospitals.

Finally, and perhaps the most sophisticated of the snipers shooting down physician-owned hospitals is the ACA. This is better known as "Obamacare," or the term that we love to talk about in the office break room, regardless of whether or not we've even read the thing. Section 6001 of this federal statute expands on the Stark Laws by prohibiting future physician investment and capping existing physician investment in hospitals, therefore establishing an immediate cap on physician ownership. When this act was signed into law in March 2010, existing physician-owned hospitals were allowed to continue to operate, but they have essentially been prevented from expanding their capacity with very few exceptions. And, as long as the ACA continues to be upheld, new physician-owned hospitals wishing to be paid with Medicare dollars are no more.

First, I want to make one thing clear. I'm not anti-EVERYTHING with Obamacare. In fact, if you are reading this, Mr. President, I'd love the opportunity to sit down with you and share ideas, because I actually like some of yours. But, I am anti-section 6001, because with it, you are crushing the very entity actually capable of reinstating value back into healthcare.

THE VALUE OF PHYSICIAN-OWNED HOSPITALS

If you are already convinced that I could own a hospital as a physician businessman that would provide you more value than a bureaucratic tanker ship, then just skip this section and close the book. No, scratch that. Actually, keep reading anyway because the end is near and the view from the top will be worth the extra climb.

In fact, I don't even want you to just take my word for it. Critics would argue that my assumptions are arrogant, so fine, disregard them. Instead, I'd rather you look at how the existing physician-owned hospitals have performed since the passing of Obamacare, and this requires us to learn one last vocabulary word, something known as the Hospital Value-based Purchasing Program (HVBP).

The HVBP is outlined in section 3001 of the ACA, but I'll summarize it more simply for you here. Hospitals want to get paid by Medicare for the services they provide. Medicare has agreed to provide bonuses to hospitals who meet certain standards and penalize those hospitals that don't. Under the HVBP, Medicare has already been adjusting its payments to hospitals since October 2012. The adjustments to Medicare's standard payments are fairly minimal in terms of absolute percentage points (for example, 1% or 2% up or down), but can mean hundreds of thousands of dollars to hospitals over the course of the year.

To assess whether a hospital will receive a bonus or a penalty, the HVBP has established certain criteria by which to judge hospitals. There are lots of details here, but you should just know that the variables affecting payments to hospitals for this year include categories like: (1) patient experience of care, (2) patient outcome, and (3) clinical process of care. To give you some understandable examples, patient experience encompasses those things that can be surveyed, such as how well patients feel that they were communicated with during their hospital stay by doctors and nurses, or the cleanliness of the facility. Patient outcome entails a hospital's survival rates for heart attack and pneumonia. Clinical process of care evaluates the percentage of patients admitted with heart failure that were treated with well-established guideline-based therapies.

Approximately 3,000 hospitals nationwide were eligible to participate in the HVBP and therefore received payment adjustments for the 2013 fiscal year. Of these nearly 3,000 hospitals, only about 160 were physician-owned, or roughly 5% of all the hospitals. So, tell me, how did the physician-owned underdog do? This is my favorite part of the story. Nine of the top 10 hospitals in the country, as judged by the Affordable Care Act's value-based metric, were physician-owned. In fact, 48 of the top 100 were physician-owned facilities. You ever heard of the Five-Fifty rule? Good, because I just made it up. It means that 5% of the players won 50% of the awards. Why? You want to know how this could have happened? I'll detail both sides of the argument below, but you need to hear this now: physician-owned hospitals were never the underdog; in fact, they were the overwhelming favorite all along! The ACA and its HVBP had created a new "game" with new rules that no one had ever played before. And, physician-owned hospitals are always better able to adapt to a new game than their tanker ship competitors. Tugboats are just more steerable in a dynamic environment, and medicine is as dynamic as it gets. The physician-owned hospitals should have been expected to blow everybody else away, and they did.

Most of your members of Congress, however, never saw this one coming. When you clip the wings of an eagle only to watch it soar higher, how can you explain yourself? Well, you convince yourself that the winner merely gamed the system despite making none of its rules. You argue that the physician-owned hospitals somehow picked only the "best" patients to treat at their facilities. You note that their patient population was overall wealthier, less sick, and underwent more elective than emergent procedures. You cite your research suggesting that increased utilization occurs in physician ownership models and then you extrapolate this data to suggest that unnecessary procedures are being performed at these facilities.

Yet, advocates for physician-owned hospitals would counter just as strongly by explaining how tugboats can better direct resources to optimize patient care. Physician-owned facilities might more commonly have single-bed private rooms, interactive TVs that allow patients to order food from outside restaurants, and a myriad of other things to make for an improved patient experience. Physician-owned facilities are frequently specialty centers with a narrow focus of care, potentiating the ability to provide a smaller scope of services with more precision and higher value. Moreover, if procedures are being done inappropriately at these facilities, why aren't medical liability attorneys swarming their doorsteps? Why are commercial insurance companies, who scrutinize every physician decision, actually steering patients toward these facilities because of their efficiencies?

No matter which side that you are on, the fact remains that the patients who showed up to these physician-owned hospitals, for whatever reason, received more measurable value in their healthcare. I find it hard to believe that anyone else, wealthy or poor, healthy or sick, would have not felt the same way.

CHAPTER 10:

Onward & Upward

"DO OR DO NOT. THERE IS NO TRY."

—YODA

I was still finishing up my medical training when the Affordable Care Act (ACA) was passed into law, effectively capping new physician ownership in hospitals. Therefore, owning my own hospital to create value for my government-funded Medicare patients is not an option at this time. The possibility might resurface again in the future, but I can't count on things that require time traveling. I must live in the here and now.

For me, that means I will focus on my private practice clinic. I can better control the value of healthcare that you receive there. I can hire the best staff, technicians, and employees, and if I fail at doing this, you can tell me about it, and I'll start again until I get it right. When you need a medical study or test that falls within my area of expertise, I'll have that service readily available for you in my own office. You will have as much of a one-stop shop of convenience that I can provide. If you still elect to use your insurance to pay for testing, you may have to meet your carrier's demands by coming in on more than one day (some insurers will not pay for more than one test on the same day). However, if that's the case, you really should demand more value from your insurance company, go find another one, or start seeing your insurance differently like I mentioned in Chapter 7. You must become just as proactive in search of value as I will be in providing it.

The only issue that will befall you is if you become extremely ill and need to find a hospital, because I just can't guarantee your value there right now. And, as you have already learned, all those seals of approval on the hospital billboard don't guarantee it either. I think that if I become really sick, I'll probably head to the Mayo Clinic in Rochester, Minnesota. I'm going to make sure that they are on my "when disaster strikes" insurance plan. I'm sure that there are a few other places like them out there, perhaps the Cleveland Clinic, that would provide you equal value. I wish you the best of luck finding those places. As for me, I'm headed to the Mayo Clinic because I've just always been impressed with their understanding of value. It's one of the few places that you can actually get through to a human being when you call the number that's easily visible on their website. It's almost as if they actually want you to call them. Imagine that? Customer service in healthcare. Find a place that understands this and you'll be all right.

My ultimate goal, however, is to keep you healthy enough in my clinic that I reduce your need for these large hospital systems. And, since you are well-versed by now, you'll recognize this as being helpful, mainly because the majority of these mega-systems are finding it harder and harder to demonstrate their value to you anyway. There probably will come a time, however, that you will need an elective medical procedure. Perhaps, your profound progressing fatigue is being caused by a heart rate that never gets above 40 beats per minute, and you need a heart pacemaker. It would be nice if I could provide this service to you in a cost-effective manner without you ever needing to enter into a larger hospital facility. What if you even need a heart catheterization, also known as an angiogram? Due to improved technologies, these types of procedures can be safely done on most patients as an outpatient day procedure. And, the good news for you is that I'm still allowed to perform these office-based procedures in my own building or something known as an Ambulatory Surgical Center.

THE HEART & VASCULAR CENTER

An Ambulatory Surgical Center (ASC) is really just a facility, separate in location from a doctor's office, geared toward patient procedures that do not require an overnight stay in a hospital bed. Most ASCs will have physician ownership, as they have been able to remain exempt from Stark Laws and the other legislative efforts previously outlined. They were originally started by physicians who wished to provide timely, convenient, and comfortable procedural services to patients in their communities, and they've become popular because they've enabled patients to avoid frequently impersonal venues like regular hospitals for certain procedures.

If I were to build an ASC, or even just an office-based procedure center, I'd call it The Heart & Vascular Center. It would be a state-of-the-art facility because I would take pride in anything that I could call my own. Don't worry, my facility would have all the same certifications as the local hospital, which as I've already told you, do not prove anything about its quality. However, I can guarantee that my facility would provide you added value, and I'll give you an example as to why.

Let's presume that you are 65 years old and have government-funded Medicare as your insurer. You've been having some concerning cardiac symptoms and you need a heart catheterization, or coronary angiogram, which is the procedure that I was talking to you about earlier. You have two options. You can have the procedure performed at the local hospital or at The Heart & Vascular Center. I'll be your doctor and perform your procedure at either place, but I can really only control your entire experience at The Heart & Vascular Center.

The Heart & Vascular Center is newly constructed, on the top floor of a medical office building with great views of the city. Its office staff, nurses, and technicians who will assist with your experience are well-trained and friendly. In fact, most of them previously worked at the large local hospital but also became frustrated dealing with a tanker ship and sought more job satisfaction in an innovative and value-driven environment. Equipment is new and updated at The Heart & Vascular Center. Floors are spotless and the overall feel is modern. You arrive only 60 minutes before the start of your procedure to check-in, and like a well-oiled machine in motion, you are quickly registered by the front desk, your pre-procedure blood work is obtained, an IV is placed, and you are further prepped by the nursing staff for your procedure. Technology abounds as handheld electronic tablets (for example, iPads) show you images of what to expect during your procedure, and then post-procedure, in the recovery room, the same devices enable the physician to review with you the findings of your procedure and the treatment strategy being recommended.

The local hospital also has a heart catheterization lab where your procedure can be performed. It's located on the ground floor, or maybe the second floor, of a tanker ship. The floor is still shiny, but the environment looks a bit older. Staff are friendly, but they ask you to arrive two or three hours prior to your procedure to check-in, because the machine moves more slowly in this overly bureaucratic environment. Modern technology is found somewhere within these walls, but it's much less visible to you throughout your experience there. You actually liked the thought of being able to see images of your heart on an iPad screen. In some odd way, this helped you better understand what's going on with your body.

Regardless, you end up having your procedure performed, and after recovering, you return home. Time passes as you ponder your overall experience undergoing the heart catheterization. Ultimately, the bill for that procedure arrives in the mail. It's the year 2014. Medicare has a standard fee schedule for this type of procedure, but believe it or not, the fee schedule for the same procedure changes depending on where it is performed. For example, for your heart catheterization in the hospital, Medicare is billed $2,587 from the hospital and $311 from your physician. You have a standard Medicare policy, without secondary insurance, which means that you are responsible for 20% of the total $2,898 billed to Medicare for your procedure at the local hospital. Your portion amounts to $580, or about half what you recently just paid to fix your car's air conditioning system. All things considered, not a bad price to pay in order for a potentially life-threatening condition to be recognized in time for successful surgical treatment.

Oh, but wait, I forgot. You elected to have your procedure done at The Heart & Vascular Center instead of the local hospital, because your best friend next door said his experience at The Heart & Vascular Center was outstanding. As mentioned above, Medicare has a different fee schedule for a heart catheterization done at this type of facility. The Heart & Vascular Center bills Medicare only $694, because truthfully they can perform the entire case in a more cost-effective manner. Your physician's bill to Medicare remains the same at $311. Of course, you will still be responsible for your standard 20%, which comes to a grand total of $201 for your procedure at The Heart & Vascular Center.

The game of numbers is clearly straightforward: $580 at the local hospital or $201 at The Heart & Vascular Center. You seemingly have two choices for the same procedure, but in all honesty, only one provides you utmost value. Essentially, The Heart & Vascular Center is upgrading your room to the Ritz-Carlton for a price that is 65% less than the Holiday Inn. I've said it once, but I'll say it again. Physician-owned facilities aren't the underdog, they are the overwhelming favorite in a value-based system. My town needs one of these places desperately. My patients deserve one. In fact, I should build one when I'm done writing this book.

ALL FOR ONE AND ONE FOR VALUE

I've made every attempt to bring you ultimate transparency in healthcare. From what I've told you, you may be wondering why I don't just hang up my private practice and implement an exit strategy. I actually could be making a better salary at this moment as an employed physician. I would even be seeing less patients in that type of model and punch more of an 8 a.m. to 6 p.m. clock. Maybe, I could be an average physician administrator for a large healthcare system and actually learn to enjoy drinking coffee at the meetings. But, I think it would be hard for me to sleep on a tanker ship. I always have the option to remain in private practice and sever my connection with government-funded insurers like Medicare and Medicaid. This would relieve some of the administrative and unnecessary documentation burden that their relationship forces upon me. But, to be honest, this seems like an easy way out, and I'm up for more of a challenge.

I know that I'm idealistic, but I actually think that I can save the system, and I mean the entire system, even the government-funded one. I can't do it alone, or maybe I actually can, if those federal statutes would just allow me to have more personal ownership of healthcare. You take more pride in things that you own anyway. That's the whole business concept of vested interest which ultimately drives value. Remember, physician owners initially started getting into the healthcare business to provide better patient care and improve efficiencies of care, not for the money. In the meantime, I'll keep meandering the land mines that are trying to blow me out of private practice. You call up your members of Congress and then make an impact by voting for anything that you see is returning value back to healthcare. And, trust me, that's not going to be anything that resembles a bureaucratic tanker ship. Like Dr. Oz, I've got a group of people who can give you hope again, and that group is made up of physician businessmen and businesswomen. Wish us godspeed.

About Green Publishing House, LLC

Green Publishing House is a Limited Liability Company dedicated to the production and global distribution of scholarly, peer-reviewed, academic books and high quality general interest trade books. Green Publishing House partners with numerous distributors to deliver valued books across multiple platforms (digital and print) at competitive costs.

The central mission of Green Publishing House is to deliver high quality digital textbooks and trade books to readers at low prices. Going digital is not only environmentally responsible and less expensive to readers, but it also offers our clients the opportunity to receive up-to-date scholarly resources on a moment's notice from millions of locations worldwide.

Although the number of digital readers is growing every year, because everyone may not have access to the internet and eBook readers, and because some individuals, book reviewers, and libraries may prefer hard copy texts, the company also offers print copies of its books. To remain loyal to its central mission, however, the company encourages the purchase of digital versions of its books, and cheerfully donates a portion of the revenue it receives from its print copy sales to educational and charitable institutions.